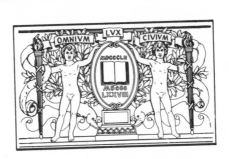

The VD Epidemic

The

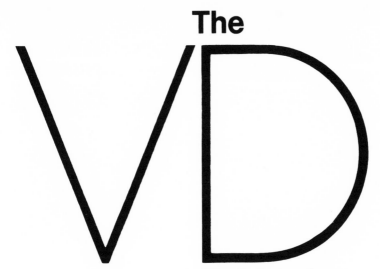

VD

Epidemic

**How It Started,
Where It's Going, and
What To Do
About It**

Louis Lasagna

Temple University Press

Philadelphia

Temple University Press, Philadelphia 19122
© 1975 by Louis Lasagna
All rights reserved
Published 1975
Printed in the United States of America

International Standard Book Number: 0-87722-041-7
Library of Congress Catalog Card Number: 74-29475

*To my children
and all other
young people,
on whom the future
depends*

"But do not hope to see the end of the scourge that is afflicting you. This disease shall be eternal. . . . Apollo has sworn it by the Styx and by immutable Destiny."

From *Syphilis,* by Hieronymus Fracastorius

Contents

Illustrations

Preface

This book owes its genesis to a suggestion from Marcia Magill, who believed the time ripe for a successor to the 1937 classic *Shadow on the Land*. My original reaction was one of doubt. I had learned a bit about venereal diseases during my association with Dr. J. Earle Moore at Hopkins, especially in editing with him the *Journal of Chronic Diseases*, and my job as a clinical pharmacologist required me to have some interest in most aspects of therapeutics, but I was hardly a VD expert. Indeed, I had not even been enterprising enough ever to contract the diseases.

But the problem was obviously an important one, and the more I read the more interested and involved I became. The advent of several recent books on VD gave me some pause, but a reading of them left me unsatisfied. None seemed quite right—they were either too short, or too long, or too superficial, or too scholarly, or not enough fun to read. The reader will have to judge whether I have overcome these deficiencies in the pages that follow.

A special vote of thanks is due Ruth Kimmerer and Kris Wemett for their labors over my handwriting in typing the many drafts and the final manuscript.

The VD Epidemic

The Monster Revives

"As a result of antibiotic therapy, gonorrhea has almost passed from the scene as an important clinical and public health entity." These words were written in 1949 by Dr. John F. Mahoney, the man whose medical team had, six years earlier, shown that penicillin could cure syphilis.

Most authorities agreed. Paul O'Leary, the distinguished editor of the *AMA Archives of Dermatology and Syphilology,* dropped the phrase "and Syphilology" from the title in 1955. Dr. J. Earle Moore, one of the internationally famous students of venereal disease, went even further. The journal he had edited for years, the *American Journal of Venereal Diseases,* was scrapped and the *Journal of Chronic Diseases* started in its place. His world-famous VD clinic at the Johns Hopkins Hospital became a Chronic Disease Clinic, since syphilis seemed to be disappearing as an important public health problem as a consequence of progress in its treatment.

Syphilology, never terribly prominent anyway in medical school curricula, was even further deemphasized. Whereas Sir William Osler had taught that "he who knows syphilis, knows medicine" (1), doctors be-

1

gan to be graduated with little knowledge of the disease, and often without having seen a chancre. Training programs for young physicians interested in becoming VD specialists fell by the wayside.

On January 28, 1956, the Board of Commissioners of the Joint Commission on Accreditation of Hospitals dropped routine admission blood tests for syphilis as a requirement for hospital accreditation. Many authorities began to question whether required premarital blood tests were not a pointless nuisance, a meaningless relic.

Federal appropriations for VD control fell from a $17 million high to $9.8 million in 1953 and $3 million in 1955. Despite the cutback in funds and in national interest in VD, the rate for primary and secondary syphilis dropped to 6.2 cases per 100,000 population in 1953 —one-tenth of the figure a decade earlier—and then to 3.8 per 100,000 in 1957 (2). The Rapid Treatment Centers that had been set up throughout the country were closed.

Then the bubble of optimism and smug satisfaction burst. In 1958 the number of reported cases of gonorrhea and infectious syphilis in the United States began to rise. In 1959, there were 237,000 cases of gonorrhea reported to health officials. By 1969 the level had reached 494,000 (3). Since there is an enormous amount of underreporting, the actual number of cases in that year was estimated at 1,800,000, an incidence of 900 per 100,000 population. (As we shall see later, even these figures are probably lower than the true ones.)

Nor was the phenomenon restricted to this country. Gonorrhea in England and Wales in 1969 was at the highest level ever recorded (4), up 14 percent over the preceding year and surpassing the previous peak year of 1946, when the population was reacting to the stresses of the recent war and demobilization. The

Swedes reported a gonorrhea rate of 485 per 100,000 (4). The figures for 1970 were even higher—rates in Denmark and Canada showed a 15 percent rise over 1969; for Canada the figure was twice what it had been in 1960. Projected worldwide figures were placed at 4 million cases of syphilis and 15 million cases of gonorrhea.

In 1971 the *New York Times* reported on a talk given at a meeting of the American Social Health Association. It was estimated that over a half million Americans were suffering from undetected syphilis and "are in urgent need of skilled medical attention" (5). Twenty-four million dollars of federal funds for VD control were called for.

In Atlanta, Georgia, the results of a three-year program of screening for gonorrhea revealed that, of 740,446 women surveyed, 8.9 percent were positive for the disease; 80 percent of these were asymptomatic. Of all the reportable communicable diseases, gonorrhea had become number one in the United States, ahead of scarlet fever and other streptococcal diseases (6). Syphilis was third. By 1972, it was estimated that one new case of gonorrhea was being acquired in the United States every fifteen seconds around the clock.

Australia reported VD to be assuming epidemic proportions, rising at the rate of 10 to 15 percent a year; gonorrhea had displaced infectious hepatitis as the most highly reported infectious disease, although experts there in obstetrics-gynecology and preventive medicine estimated that no more than 5 to 7 percent of cases were being reported. Newborn babies with gonorrhea were being seen in increasing numbers. The practice of applying a silver nitrate solution prophylactically to children's eyes at the time of birth having been discontinued, babies were developing gonococcal infection of the eyes. Medical authorities took some comfort from the fact that at least this way they were able to tell that the mother had the disease and needed treatment.

Editorials in the British journal *Lancet* began to call attention to the growing seriousness of the venereal plague: "Gonorrhea is now the commonest infectious disease which is curable by antibiotic therapy" (7). The disease was said to be second only to the common cold in incidence. There was a great increase in the incidence of gonococcal infection of the fallopian tubes (the ones that lead from the ovaries to the uterus); in some American hospitals as many as one of every five gynecological inpatients had this infection, and about 20 percent of these women were sterile (8). In Seattle, the serious complications of gonorrhea—such as arthritis, heart valve infection, and meningitis—were diagnosed with increasing frequency. A report from the Mayo Clinic stated that rectal gonorrhea was proving particularly hard to treat; one from Memphis found an increase in symptomless gonorrhea. Everywhere, the medical profession was being warned that the magnitude of the disaster was even greater than it seemed.

What had brought about the epidemic of the sixties and seventies? What had produced the complacency of the 1950's? William J. Brown, formerly chief of the Veneral Disease Branch of the Communicable Disease Center of the Public Health Service, has said: "As a disease *control* program approaches the end-point of eradication, it is the *program* rather than the disease which is more likely to be eradicated" (1). The reasons are not mysterious. In the case of syphilis and gonorrhea, the continuing and apparently projectable decline in the diseases fostered the illusion that the problems were headed for inevitable extinction.

A second factor was the low mortality rate. VD was not killing more than a few thousand Americans a year and thus did not qualify as a major cause of mortality. It is fascinating to remember, however, that the same could be said for poliomyelitis, which in its peak years in the United States never afflicted more than 40 people per 100,000, and averaged one death per 100,000 per year. Yet effective publicity, sparked by President Roosevelt's paralysis and the National Foundation's imaginative efforts, mobilized national concern to a degree unrelated to the numerical aspects of the problem and eventually eliminated the disease, to all intents and purposes.

A third reason lay in the epidemiologic aspects of VD control. As a communicable disease decreases in incidence, cases become harder to find. As difficulty in case-finding increases, the process becomes more expensive and demands more refined techniques. Enthusiasm quite naturally flags as everyone has to work harder and harder and spend more and more money for fewer and fewer returns.

Many other factors contributed to the resurgence of VD. The advent of penicillin eliminated the need for prolonged arsenical treatment (see Chapter 5) and shifted the focus of VD therapy from the public clinic to the private doctor's office. The greater efficacy of the new antibiotics should have been a boon; instead, it led to all sorts of new problems. For some, easier treatment decreased the fear of syphilis. Physicians unversed in VD tended to be less accurate in their diagnosis, less adept at treatment, and almost totally unfitted for surveillance of contacts and follow-up of their own patients. The private doctor's concern about the confidentiality of his relationship to his patient increased the amount of underreporting. Furthermore, the gonococcus (like many other bacteria) began to develop resistance, first to the sulfa drugs and then to penicillin.

Sex mores, never static, were changing at an accelerated rate. A variety of cultural forces have been blamed for what many feel to be an increasing promiscuity in Western cultures. Everything has been indicted from the Viet Nam war and the atom bomb to motels, "simplified clothing," and the zippered fly. They are easy to cite, but difficult to quantify.

Young people have become a prime target for criticism, and one cannot deny that there is a lot of VD among teenagers. In Los Angeles, a survey of one thousand males aged fifteen to sixty elicited the interesting fact that over half of them had contracted gonorrhea for the first time by the age of sixteen (3). Six-year-old boys have been found to have VD, and even younger girls who have been sexually molested by older males are seen in hospital emergency rooms, suffering from gonococcal vulvovaginitis. Sweden's rise in VD has been greatest in the fifteen to nineteen year old age group, although the U.S. figures show the greatest number of cases of both gonorrhea and syphilis in the twenty to twenty-four year old group, with a lot of disease, however, also in the fifteen to nineteen and the twenty-five to twenty-nine year groups, and a great increase in the incidence of syphilis in the age group thirty to forty-nine (3). So, VD does occur chiefly in teenagers and young adults, even if chancres have been reported in adventuresome elders of eighty-one and ninty-one years of age.

Is there more promiscuity than before? It's hard to be sure, although the available data suggest earlier and more frequent premarital sex and more extramarital activity. Part of this can be traced to the advent of new contraceptive techniques. The "Pill" and intrauterine devices do not just decrease the likelihood of pregnancy; they also lower the barriers (both psychological and esthetic) to sexual intercourse. Their replacement of the diaphragm as the major contraceptive technique has been harmful in other ways: diaphragm jelly is a partial barrier against VD; gonorrhea can be more serious when acquired by a woman with an IUD in her uterus; and the changes in the vagina that occur when one takes the Pill are thought by some to facilitate growth of the gonococcus. Men and women of all ages who might previously have been dissuaded from sexual adventures by the inconvenience of mechanical devices have been liberated by the newer techniques, although sometimes by paying a considerable price. The young girl who could have avoided unwanted sex in the old days now has no convincing excuse and may find herself not only psychologically traumatized by undesired intercourse, but infected as well.

The rise of the Pill and the IUD has been accompanied by a decline in the popularity of the condom. While penile sheaths can prevent the transmission of VD only to a limited degree and are not going to be much help if a lot of foreplay goes on prior to their donning, condoms properly used are at least a partial impediment to the spread of VD.

The young people who have been led, by their disenchantment with what they interpret as the cynical materialism and hypocrisy of our society, to become vagrants and members of communes with numerous readily available sex partners are often found to suffer from malnutrition, hepatitis, and venereal disease. The latter problem has become so severe that anti-VD campaigns have been waged by the young people themselves and by the volunteer physicians who minister to their emotional and medical needs.

The wars of recent vintage have also received their share of blame, since martial conflict and postwar problems have over the years been associated with outbreaks of VD. Past increases in VD seem to have occurred immediately after a war, rather than in times of mobilization or combat, but this situation seems to be changing, in part because it has become increasingly difficult to differentiate war from nonwar periods and in part because the well-organized opportunities for traffic with prostitutes in places like Southeast Asia defy comparisons with older wars.

One possibly important lesson for us from Army experience, however, lies in the history of legislative penalties. In 1926 an Act of Congress was drafted to punish armed forces members who contracted VD. In 1944 it was repealed, since it seemed to cause more harm than good by encouraging concealment and thus fostering the spread of disease.

Prostitution has been a significant contributor to VD over the centuries. Restricting whorehouses to an area of a city, or inspecting prostitutes for disease, has never really achieved much, and today's call-girls, "cruisers," semipro housewives, and amateurs have widely expanded the opportunities for recreational sex. So has the increasing trend toward urbanization, which makes casual contacts easier and less noticeable than in small towns, not only because of less scrutiny from one's neighbors but because of the lessened importance of family units and the greater cultural acceptance of promiscuity. A former medical colleague of mine was once asked by one of the country's most publicized lawyers to dine with him to discuss the possibility of the doctor's testifying in a malpractice suit. Arriving at the hotel, the physician joined the lawyer at his table and found three gorgeous call girls also in attendance. The doctor was offered his pick for a quick tumble in a readily available bedroom "before we get down to business."

The large city also has a greater tolerance for homosexuality, an increasingly important phenomenon. (Dr. N. Fiumara, a Massachusetts VD expert, has said that the average heterosexual patient names four contacts;

the average homosexual names ten.) The major VD threat comes from the male, rather than the female, homosexual. Lesbians are less likely to be promiscuous than gay men, and the greatest source of infection is the young (under thirty), highly promiscuous, sexually versatile, white-collar or professional homosexual male.

We are also, as a society, paying a price for increased mobility. The average length of residence at one address is said to be about five years. Cheap air travel, package holidays, and speedy jets allow men and women to rival the merchant seamen of old, although a 1948 U.S. Public Health Study of eighty unselected seamen recorded that they could boast of sexual intercourse with 615 persons in 112 ports in 45 countries— a mark for today's jumbo jet devotee to shoot at (9). A 1971 World Health Organization report alleged that 50 percent of venereal infections in the Scandinavian countries were acquired abroad (4).

Finally, one must add to the causes of the VD epidemic the unenlightened public attitudes toward these diseases. At one extreme there is hypocrisy and secrecy. In Los Angeles, it is illegal to teach about VD in the public school system without parental consent, despite the fact that surveys indicate that young people are abysmally ignorant about VD. At the other extreme, there is apathy and nonchalance. In a British VD clinic, 27 percent of men with gonorrhea had had the infection before—17 percent once, 5 percent twice, and 5 percent three times. Nine percent had had it twice in one year. Indeed, Fleming, the discoverer of penicillin, is alleged to have said, "We have made it possible to catch gonorrhea three times a week." Dr. F. L. Roberts, a Memphis VD expert, wrote the following pessimistic letter to the *Journal of the American Medical Association:*

We cannot get 80% of our patients back in one week even when we pay them $10 for the return visit, which we do on some research projects; it would be impossible to get any of them back for ten consecutive days. . . . We treat 12,000 to 13,000 cases of gonorrhea a year. After three to seven days, we are unable to rule out reinfection in our clients and have no faith whatever that the patients will take the drugs outside the clinic. (We have found capsules of tetracycline in the waiting room waste-baskets.) . . . Since the days of the Old Testament writers, gonorrhea has been with us. The gonococcus is almost as adaptable as the cockroach and will probably become resistant to any drug (10).

The picture is not all gloomy, to be sure. Despite the worldwide increase in early syphilis beginning in the 1950's, there has been a sustained decrease in congenital syphilis in most countries. Even the exceptions of Africa and Asia may be suffering from confusion of VD with such nonvenereal diseases as yaws, to be described in Chapter 4. The so-called nonvenereal treponematoses of childhood, which are bacteriologically related to syphilis and which afflict the rural populations of developing countries, have been decreased to an astonishing degree by WHO mass campaigns in forty-five countries, using injections of long-acting penicillins.

Not only have late and congenital syphilis fallen steadily in the United States since 1941, but so have the so-called minor venereal diseases (like chancroid, lymphogranuloma venereum, and so on). Deaths from syphilis have dropped from over fourteen thousand a year in 1940 to about two thousand, although satisfaction over that achievement is tainted by the knowledge that only tuberculosis, of all the reportable infectious diseases, kills more Americans each year (3).

So, we have made both national and international

progress in some VD areas, only to see disaster strike on other fronts. Can we correct the reverses? A lot depends on whether we face up to the task. For 1971, $75 million in expenditures were authorized by the Communicable Disease Amendments of 1970, but Washington financed only $2 million worth. Fiscal 1972 had an authorization of $90 million, but only a small fraction was actually spent. The Nixon administration, with its generally low estimate of the importance of medical funding, did not help the situation any, and the current gloomy economic scene does not augur well for federal health programs. In any case, a steady, serious approach is needed, year in and year out, not a roller-coaster philosophy.

When will we stop playing games with VD? When will we stop talking about it and actually pay for the facilities and the personnel to eradicate it? It is a pity that we lack a powerful and effective lobby against VD. Until the people wake, money will continue to be spent for military weapons that kill man rather than for medical weapons against the microorganisms of syphilis and gonorrhea, for projects to put a few astronauts on the moon rather than for programs to cure the infected millions here on earth.

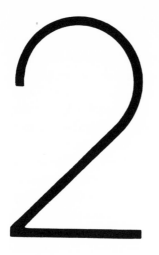

The Beginnings of VD

No country wants credit for the origin of syphilis. When European chroniclers began to pay attention to the disease toward the end of the fifteenth century, there was only a sort of reverse national pride in disowning the malady—the English and the Turks called it the French disease, the Persians blamed it on the Turks, the Flemish and Dutch referred to it as the Spanish pox, the French called it the Italian or Neapolitan disease, the Italians blamed it either on the Spanish or the French, the Portuguese termed it the Castilian disease, the Spaniards called it the disease of the Isle of Española (where Columbus had been), the Russians thought of it as a Polish ailment, and the Poles gave credit to the Germans.

Where did syphilis first occur? We know that a severe form of syphilis, in epidemic form, swept over Europe, and possibly from there to other continents, starting around 1500. One major historical hypothesis has been that the natives of America repaid their ravaging European conquerors by exposing them for the first time to a disease that had long existed in the New World. The evidence for this is in several forms.

To begin with, the European literature before Columbus seems devoid of descriptions that might fit our modern concepts of the disease. In 1495 the Holy Roman Emperor Maximilian issued an edict referring to the "evil pocks which had never occurred before nor been heard of in the memory of man." He called it a punishment sent by God for blasphemy. Then, bones have been found in many parts of North and South America that seem to some experts unquestionably syphilitic, whereas pre-Columbian syphilitic skeletons from Europe are almost nonexistent. (There are a few, but none is definitively accepted as both pre-Columbian and syphilitic.) Finally, the severity of the disease as it was first recognized in Europe is considered evidence in favor of its being a new disease there. Infections appearing de novo in nonimmune populations are notoriously more dangerous than diseases that have been experienced before by a people, and for the first fifty years syphilis in Europe was not infrequently a rapidly fatal affliction, in contrast to its slower, more benign nature today.

But this Columbian theory has not gone unquestioned. Aleš Hrdlička, a distinguished anthropologist, has offered the opinion that not one of the thousands of pre-Columbian skulls and skeletons found in America can be thoroughly authenticated as syphilitic (3). Nor does one see syphilitic lesions depicted in American pre-Columbian sculpture.

The leprosy of ancient times—or at least part of it—may have been syphilis. The reasons for thinking this are several. First, the old accounts sometimes use phrases such as "venereal" or "congenital" leprosy. Neither adjective is applicable to leprosy—at least as we know it today—but both apply beautifully to syphilis. Second, the leprosy of old was thought to be highly contagious, yet today leprosy is a disease that is usually acquired only after prolonged and intimate contact with lepers. Third, the Saracen's Ointment, brought back by the returning Crusaders in the eleventh to fourteenth centuries, contained mercury and was supposed to be efficacious for "leprosy." Again, this story is more appropriate if the ointment were applied to syphilitic lesions; leprosy is not thought to respond to mercury, but the one possibly beneficial effect of mercury in syphilis is that achieved by local application.

Hieronymus Fracastorius (also referred to as Jerome Fracastor, or Girolamo Fracastoro)—of whom more later—knew that the majority of people acquired syphilis by contagion, but he doubted that it would have spread so fast in so many places if it had just been brought back to Naples by a single small fleet of Spanish ships (3). Some Oriental scholars believe that the Chinese knew the symptoms of secondary syphilis by at least 2600 B.C., recognized the existence of congenital syphilis, and knew the difference between gonorrhea and syphilis, although others are skeptical about the possibility of precise diagnosis in a period that lacked laboratory aids.

Hackett has hypothesized that the spirochetal organisms causing syphilis hark back to an evolutionary offshoot of a main stem of microorganisms that infected animals only until 15,000 B.C. (3). From this main line, he believes the various treponemal diseases arose separately. Other students of evolution argue that the nonvenereal disease yaws (see Chapter 4) came off the "animal" branch of the family tree about 10,000 B.C. and that all other spirochetal diseases derived from it. These speculations were strengthened considerably in 1963 by the discovery of a treponemal disease in African monkeys so mild that except for a slight enlargement of lymph nodes behind the knees the health of the monkeys seemed almost unimpaired. It is argued that the evolution of treponemal diseases was affected by both climate and clothing—cooler temperatures changing the infective power of the bugs and also forcing man to acquire clothing. The latter first changed the mode of transmission from skin to oral contact—or so the story goes—and then, as still more clothing was acquired, to venereal contact (around 3000 B.C.).

In 1971, some new evidence appeared. Neanderthal skeletons show bony abnormalities that have been thought to be caused by rickets. Dr. D. J. M. Wright, a British venereologist, suggested that they are also compatible with congenital syphilis (11). These changes— the so-called "Olympian brow," for example—affected not only the skull of the original Neanderthal man, but also those of contemporary adult and child skeletons found in other parts of Europe. Other features compatible with syphilis are the relative depression of the bridge of the nose ("saddle nose"), and the dental abnormalities of these skulls. The curved long bones, especially the backward curve of the femur, were what first made the famous pathologist Virchow opine that Neanderthal man was just *Homo sapiens* with rickets. But syphilitic inflammation of the bone produces the same sort of changes and would in addition account for Neanderthal bones being so short and stout.

Wright argues further that if Neanderthal man was so rachitic, Neanderthal woman should have had great difficulties in delivering her babies, since her pelvic bones would have been deformed. But no such pelvic changes have ever been noted in Neanderthal skeletons. He concludes that the observed skeletal changes provide a link between monkey treponematosis and our present human disease.

Even granted the validity of this second theory, one still has to explain the explosive character of sixteenth-century European syphilis. We have to fall back either

on substantial increases in travel across national bound-
aries, abetted by "free-thinking" and changes in mores
as a result of the wars and the Black Death, or postulate
a sudden mutation of the syphilitic organism into a
more virulent strain.

But let us return to the history of syphilis. A Spanish
physician named Dias de Isla was in practice in Bar-
celona in 1493, when Columbus's first expedition to the
New World returned. In his writings, Dias alleges that
"the serpentine disease" was unknown prior to this
date and that it was introduced to the inhabitants of the
city by Columbus's crewmen on their return from Española (2). From that point on, knowledge of syphilis as
a phenomenon spread rapidly—woodcuts as early as
1496 portrayed the skin lesions, and in a sixteenth-century representation of the impediments of armies one
can see depicted the "triumph of the high and mighty
Dame Syphilis, Queen of the Fountain of Love" (2).

More than forty sixteenth-century physicians wrote
treatises on the disease, the most famous being Fracastorius, who provided a name for the scourge in a poem
about an afflicted, impious shepherd named Syphilus.
Although Fracastorius had developed an early theory
of the microbic origin of infections, several centuries
were to elapse before the germ theory of disease received experimental support and general scientific acceptance. Nevertheless, the contribution of sexual intercourse to the transmission of syphilis was recognized
almost from the start. The entity of congenital syphilis
was also soon appreciated.

At first syphilis was to a certain degree differentiated
from gonorrhea, but later the two diseases became confused with each other. Helping no little in engendering
confusion in this regard was John Hunter, a famous
eighteenth-century English anatomist. In an excess of
experimental zeal, Hunter inoculated himself with

gonorrheal pus from a patient who also had syphilis and erroneously concluded that syphilis and gonorrhea were the same disease.

In the nineteenth century, the two ailments were more clearly distinguished, primarily because of the observations of theFrench school of syphilographers. One of these, Philippe Ricord, was not only a fine clinician but a great wit. America's own great physician-wit, Oliver Wendell Holmes, called him "the Voltaire of pelvic literature—a skeptic as to the morality of the race in general, who would have submitted Diana to treatment with his mineral specifics and ordered a course of blue pills for the vestal virgins" (12). Ricord believed that venereal diseases had always plagued mankind: "In the beginning, God created the heavens, the earth, man and venereal diseases" (13). He epitomized the seriousness of syphilis with the aphorism "the pox is a pitiless creditor and grants grace to no one (14).

Little by little, the scientific gaps were filled in. The late complications of syphilis were gradually recognized. The causative agent was discovered by Fritz Schaudinn and Erich Hoffman in the years 1905–10. In 1906 the diagnostic Wassermann test was developed. And the first major therapeutic weapon, arsphenamine, was discovered by Paul Ehrlich in 1910.

Gonorrhea, the other major venereal disease, is thought by some to have been known to the ancient Egyptians and Assyrians and to early Chinese and Japanese civilization. The Book of Leviticus even contains a passage anticipating the now largely discredited "toilet seat" theory of the spread of venereal disease: "everything, wherever he sitteth, shall be unclean. . . . And what saddle soever he rideth upon that hath the issue shall be unclean."

The disease was given its name by Galen in the second century after Christ's birth and means "flow of seed," presumably because of the similarity between seminal ejaculate and the penile discharge so characteristic of the disease in males. The thirteenth-century physician William of Saliceto seemed aware of the venereal nature of gonorrhea, attributing the disease to retention of impurities under the male prepuce after exposure to "unclean" women and suggesting prevention by washing. One cannot be sure, however, that by "unclean" he didn't mean somebody who had leprosy or even a woman who was simply menstruating (3).

Some of the most famous physicians of centuries past (including Paracelsus and John Hunter) taught that gonorrhea was a symptom of syphilis. In 1879, however, Neisser identified the causative agent—the family of germs which is named after him also includes the cause of meningococcal meningitis—and named it the gonococcus. A few years later the organism, grown on artificial medium in pure culture, was shown to cause the disease when inoculated into the human urethra. An important step forward was the discovery in the 1880's by the obstetrician Karl Credé that the routine instillation of silver nitrate drops in the eyes of newborns would prevent gonococcal infection at that site. Eventually, the disease itself became amenable to treatment as the sulfa drugs and then penicillin were introduced in the 1930's and 1940's.

While it is clear that venereal diseases were widespread in the Western world after 1500, accurate figures as to their prevalence are impossible to obtain. Not only were there no reliable laboratory means of confirming the diagnosis for four centuries, but interest in epidemiology and public health statistics also lagged. In the nineteenth century, however, some serious attempts to quantify the prevalence of syphilis were made. On the basis of history and clinical findings alone, it was believed that at least 5 to 10 percent of the European population was syphilitic. In big cities, where prostitution was more likely to flourish, the estimates were even higher: 12 percent for Berlin and 15 percent for Paris (2). Blood testing, if available, would almost certainly have raised these already substantial figures.

Because of the records kept on military personnel, many of the figures in such records for the period 1860–1910 have been scrutinized for clues as to what might have been happening in the civilian population. For the Prussian Army, syphilis rates fell from the range of 7.5 to 9.7 per 1,000 during the 1876–1886 decade to 4 to 5.2 per 1,000 in 1910. British Army records, thought to be more reliable, showed a steady fall from 102 per 1,000 in 1890 to 20 in 1910. The U.S. Army data show fluctuations between 11 and 73 per 1,000 for the years from 1821 to 1910, with substantial rises in the wake of the Mexican, Civil, and Spanish-American Wars (2). J. Earle Moore, one of America's most famous students of venereal disease, showed that with few exceptions the major armies of the Western world experienced sizable decreases in the reported incidence and prevalence of syphilis for the 1860–1910 period. Then, during World War I, both the neutral Dutch Army and the combatant French Army reported large jumps in syphilis.

No one can say that these figures reflect, except in the crudest way, what was going on in the civilian populations of Europe, but most experts believe that the general decline cited was both real and general. Why the change? It certainly could not be attributed to control measures, nor to the essentially useless treatments then available. A more likely explanation was the rapid rise in the standard of living and in public education following the Industrial Revolution. Syphilis has never been evenly distributed in the population, tending to be more frequent in the poor and in the badly educated, perhaps because of their greater sexual activity and higher level of extramarital intercourse.

After 1910, medical science could offer blood and microscopic tests for syphilis, as well as active treatment. Scandinavian countries such as Sweden and Norway mounted public treatment and control programs and reduced the attack rate considerably. By contrast, American programs were at first weak and probably had minimal impact. In 1938 it was estimated that Americans stood one chance in ten of acquiring syphilis before they died (2). With the advent of World War II, draftee records furnished accurate information as to the prevalence of syphilis in men aged eighteen to forty (2). Blood tests were positive for syphilis in 1.8 percent of whites and 24.5 percent of blacks. Using these figures as a base, experts calculated that one in forty-two Americans had syphilis, although this average masked very real differences not only between whites and blacks, but also between different parts of the country. Rates for both races were highest in the South, for example.

In 1938, under the leadership of Surgeon General Thomas Parran, the Syphilis Control Program finally began to be effective. The reported cases of infectious syphilis dropped from a high of over 100,000 in 1947 to a low point of 6,500 in 1957 (2). The upsurge that would have been expected as a consequence of World War II was largely contained, until the changing events of the 1950's, described in Chapter 1, reversed the decline.

No historical reference to the venereal diseases can ignore the famous people that have been thought to be afflicted by these infections. The farther back one goes in history, the less reliable tend to be our guesses about the ailments of the time, but VD has been attributed to such legendary figures as Abraham, Sarah, David, Bathsheba, and Job; to Herod, Cleopatra, Julius Caesar,

Tiberius, and Commodus (Suetonius's *Lives of the Twelve Caesars* abundantly describes the sexual appetites and the homosexuality of the Roman rulers); to Charles the Fifth of France, Benvenuto Cellini, and at least three popes, Alexander VI, Julius II, and Leo X, to name only a few. Henry VIII's syphilis probably infected most of his wives, contributing in no small measure to their unfortunate obstetrical histories. Mary, the daughter of Catherine of Aragon, is thought now to have exhibited the stigmata of congenital syphilis, and it is speculated that she died when a major artery, its wall weakened by syphilis, burst. In more modern times, the list of famous personages who contracted gonorrhea, syphilis, or both has included King Edward VII, Mussolini, and Hitler.

Are these ancient accounts only of lurid interest, or do they provide a lesson for moderns? Certainly they remind us that VD is no respecter of rank, religion, or power. Today, as VD becomes an increasing problem for the well-to-do, it behooves us to recall and regret the loss to mankind inflicted by the sexual diseases. Civilization is the poorer because the brains of Nietzsche, Hugo Wolf, Edouard Manet, Dostoevski, Gluck, Donizetti, and Robert Schumann fell prey to the destructive spirochete of syphilis. The premature cutting off of their genius is not a cause for secret shame. It is a reason for public lamentation and for pledging a renewed attack on diseases that can not only shorten life but rob existence of meaning.

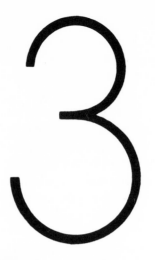

Symptoms, Sources, and Consequences

Syphilis has been called the Great Mimicker. It is an extraordinarily complex disease, with many stages, a long course (at least in some untreated individuals), and the ability to affect many parts of the body.

How does it begin? Syphilis is almost always contracted by direct transfer of the offending organism—which we shall discuss at greater length in Chapter 4—from one person to another. There must be contact between moist surfaces, and this contact is usually sexual. There are exceptions to this rule, but they are few. A physician can, for instance, acquire the disease in the process of examining a patient. The baby of an infected mother can be infected in the uterus. Dr. Evan Thomas, in his classic book on syphilis (15), tells of an octagenarian grandfather who came to clinic with a chancre on his shoulder. A little detective work explained the unusual site: he had been carrying in his arms a baby with syphilitic sores on its mouth and nose.

It is fortunate for the human race that syphilis does not spread by ordinary contact; otherwise everyone in the world would soon acquire the disease. Despite the relative unimportance of nonsexual transmission, the person with early syphilis in a highly infectious stage should certainly not be careless about the drinking vessels or towels that he uses.

The infecting spirochete—a corkscrew, spiraling organism—has to penetrate the skin or a mucous membrane (such as mouth, vagina, or rectum) to initiate the disease. Once in, it's too late to halt its growth, so that local cleansing can help only if it prevents entrance of the bug into the body.

The mischief is not recognized until the primary lesion—the chancre—appears. The interval between infection and appearance of a diagnosable lesion is variable, running between ten and ninety days. Although some men may not develop the chancre, most do sometime within three to four weeks. Women, however, have the bad luck to develop lesions in less noticeable parts of the body, so that it is quite common for female syphilitics never to be aware of the primary lesion. (The disturbing tendency for women to have less easily diagnosed VD will be encountered again when we come to gonorrhea.)

If the primary phase is skipped, either because no chancre develops or because it is not noticed, the diagnosis cannot be entertained before the sixth week of infection. The manifestations of secondary syphilis take at the very least that long to appear, and in fact usually occur in eight to sixteen weeks. The importance of this incubation period is obvious: the infected victim has a contagious disease for two to three months and doesn't know it. Blood tests—to be described in Chapter 4— can lead to a diagnosis earlier, but a person who looks and feels well is not likely to run down to the nearest VD clinic or doctor's office for a blood test.

What, actually, is a chancre? It begins as a small, indistinct, hard area which goes on to become a painless raised lesion with a flat top. Ultimately the top breaks down and becomes moist. Can you have more than one chancre at the same time? Yes, although it's much less common. While a chancre is highly suggestive in appearance, it is not so unique as to be characteristic of syphilis. The chancre can, for example, be confused with a number of other venereal diseases, such as chancroid, granuloma inguinale, and lymphogranuloma venereum. The experienced venereologist, however, has ways of discriminating between those possibilities with a reasonable degree of accuracy. Chancroid lesions and a fever blister virus known as herpes progenitalis hurt, for example; chancres do not. Syphilis is associated with enlarged but painless lymph glands in both groins; lymphogranuloma venereum also produces big groin glands, but they are usually on only one side and are painful. Granuloma inguinale is usually not a cause of enlarged lymph nodes.

Other venereal diseases are not the only sources of confusion. Cancer, scabies, injuries, drug rashes, and fungus infections can cause sores that resemble a syphilitic chancre. To separate out all these possibilities calls for clinical skill and the proper use of a variety of laboratory aids.

Aside from the chancre and enlarged glands in the area draining the chancre, there is nothing to see at this time. Since the chancre usually precedes the presence of a positive blood test, early definitive diagnosis requires that someone suspect the possibility of syphilis and that a knowledgeable person identify the spirochete by examining material from the chancre under the microscope.

The problem of diagnosis is not helped by the fact that chancres always heal themselves, even in the absence of treatment, although usually not before the secondary manifestations occur. During all this time, the spirochetes are spreading busily throughout the body. They are in the blood before one can see any lesions, and the blood is probably most infectious about the time the chancre appears. The spirochetes do not remain in the blood and lymph nodes, but invade the rest of the body.

The secondary lesions that attract attention are in the skin and mucous membranes. They are loaded with spirochetes, which probably are seeded back into the blood stream from these areas. Probably all tissues are involved at this time, but the skin and mucous membrane changes are visible while the others are not.

The primary and secondary stages have some things in common, but they differ in important ways, apart from the nature of the lesions.Unlike the primary stage, the secondary stage affects men and women similarly and blood tests are almost always positive.

Like the primary stage, the secondary can be confused with a lot of other diseases. The confusion here does not involve other venereal diseases, but rather such skin ailments as pityriasis rosea, psoriasis, lichen planus, ringworm, drug eruptions, and parasitic infestations. Secondary syphilis can also mimic such acute infectious diseases as measles, German measles, and scarlet fever.

Especially easy to mistake for secondary syphilis is infectious mononucleosis. Both are associated with sore throat, a rash, and enlarged glands, and certain of the blood tests for syphilis may be positive in mononucleosis. It is interesting that infectious mononucleosis is now thought to be most often spread by kissing that involves a good deal of tongue activity; minor epidemics have been known to afflict college communities after big dance weekends. Since Venus is the goddess of love, mononucleosis might be considered a venereal disease.

The secondary lesions of syphilis almost never itch and they never leave scars. While they can last for a year or more if untreated, they generally disappear in a few weeks or months. If untreated, a syphilitic person acquires permanent immunity to the early phases of the disease. Such a person can therefore be reinfected without developing any warning in the form of a chancre or skin or mucous membrane manifestations. By contrast, a patient whose early syphilis is adequately treated can be reinfected and develop new lesions within a few days after treatment. If a person is *inadequately* treated, he may relapse three to nine months later, either with new clinical manifestations or only with a recurrently positive blood test; such patients must be retreated.

Many patients come to medical attention with only a past history of untreated infection or a positive blood test. In the absence of any other evidence of disease, they are said to be in the latent phase. "Latent" does not mean harmless; the spirochetes may be alive in the tissues, working their mischief out of sight. This is not usually an infectious stage, although some of these patients can transmit syphilis if they donate blood, and the latent syphilitic who becomes pregnant can infect the fetus in utero.

What happens to "latent" syphilitics if untreated? At the turn of the nineteenth century, Professor Boeck of Oslo, Norway, pursued a policy of nontreatment which allowed his successors to gain some insight into the problem. Professor Boeck believed that the therapy available at that time was useless (16), so from 1891 to 1910 he withheld all treatment from 1,978 patients with primary or secondary syphilis, although he hospitalized all of them for one to twelve months—the average was 3.6 months—until all obvious traces of the disease had disappeared, so as to protect other members of the community from infection.

In 1929, his successor, Dr. E. Bruusgaard, reported a

follow-up on 473 of these (17), and from 1948 to 1951, Dr. Trygve Gjestland determined the fate of three times this number (18). Professor Boeck necessarily relied on clinical examination and the subsequent course of the disease to substantiate his diagnostic impression; darkfield microscopic examination and serologic tests were not available to him. Nevertheless, later workers do not doubt that the great majority of his patients did have syphilis.

Dr. Gjestland picked 1,404 of Boeck's original 1,978 for study, eliminating 574 foreigners and Norwegians who were not residents of Oslo so as to aid in tracing the patients and in selecting an appropriate and convenient control group for comparison. The study patients had come from the underprivileged section of society living in the east zone of Oslo; 958 were men and 446 women. At the start of Boeck's study, one half were fifteen to twenty-four years of age, a third were twenty-five to thirty-nine years old, and less than a hundred each were under fifteen or forty and over.

It is difficult to appreciate how much work and planning were involved in this Herculean effort. The investigative team scrutinized, for example, the death registers, the files of the Department of Dermatology and Venereology of the Rikshospitalet, the Oslo Bureau of Indigents, the Marriage Registry of the Central Bureau of Statistics for Oslo, the city's Population Register, and the records of the VD Divisions of the Oslo City Health Department and of the Oslo Municipal Hospital. The place of birth of each patient was studied by consulting parish ministers, sheriffs, and local population registers. The same was done for places of residence prior to the patient's settling in Oslo. Friends and relatives were sought out. Death certificates were obtained from the Oslo City Health Department and the Central Bureau of Statistics. Mental hospitals, psychiatric and neurological wards of general hospitals, and private practitioners were visited for whatever data could be garnered. At the end, there was usable information on 81.7 percent of the original 1,404, a fantastic feat considering that the interval between original study and the follow-up was at least forty years and for some patients sixty years.

What had been the medical history of all these patients? Almost a quarter of them had "relapses" within five years of discharge from the hospital, some of these patients having had multiple episodes. So-called "benign late syphilis" (this and other late manifestations will be discussed later in this chapter) occurred in about 15 percent of the patients, as early as one year and as late as forty-six years after discharge, although most showed this type of sequela by the fifteenth year.

Cardiovascular syphilis occurred in 14 percent of the men and 8 percent of the women, and appeared in no patient who had been infected prior to the age of fifteen. By contrast, central nervous system syphilis did develop in some of the infected youngsters, although not in any man infected after the age of forty. Five percent of the women and 9.4 percent of the men developed neurosyphilis.

The mortality from syphilis was twice as high in the men as in the women, although for neither sex was it an important cause of death. Approximately 90 percent of deaths were due to other diseases, such as tuberculosis, cancer, nonsyphilitic heart disease, and respiratory ailments. As of 1951, 16.1 percent of the men and 19.5 percent of the women were still alive. On the other hand, the syphilitics as a group died at earlier ages than did the population group from which they came. Clinical relapse or benign late syphilis did not appear to have prognostic significance.

What, then, can we conclude from this classic study

and the monograph of 500 pages, 83 tables, 12 figures (not to mention an appendix of 70 pages, 30 tables, and 2 figures) that it produced? It appears that 60 to 70 percent of these untreated syphilitics went through life with a minimum of inconvenience, although the final outcome for any given patient was not predictable by the baseline data at the time their infection was first diagnosed. What is completely unknown is how many new cases of syphilis they may have caused among their sexual contacts.

Let us now consider the late stages of syphilis, as well as the problems of congenital syphilis. So-called tertiary syphilis is a problem primarily for the patient; a person in this stage will rarely infect anyone else either by sexual contact or by blood donation. The one important exception is the pregnant syphilitic, who may transmit syphilis to the fetus regardless of the duration of her disease.

Late benign syphilis is so called because the lesions of this variety seldom result in physical incapacity or death, although if the characteristic "gumma" occurs in a vital organ like the brain or heart, the results can be far from benign. Gummas occur most commonly in the skin, bone, and liver and are thought to be the result of a hypersensitivity reaction to treponemal infection. The lesions may be tiny or four inches or more in diameter. To the eye, they may resemble cancer; on microscopic examination, they resemble the cheesy nodules of tuberculosis. Only rarely can one find the causative spirochete in a gumma.

In 1962, a study was performed on some Sing Sing prisoners that sheds light on the pathogenesis of gummas (19). Sixty-two volunteers were inoculated with syphilis spirochetes. Eight of the men had no previous history of syphilis; they all were infected. Twenty-six had late latent syphilis, but had been adequately treated in the past. Only ten of these developed an infection, one of them showing a gumma at the site of inoculation. Five of the prisoners had been well treated in the past for late congenital syphilis; one of these developed a gumma. The experiment proved that exogenous infection in a sensitized person can produce a gumma.

Neurosyphilis, by contrast, is a fearsome complication. It may take a variety of forms, including combinations of the major types to be described. For all types, however, the essential changes are due to an obliterative inflammation of small arteries, with associated death of nervous tissue.

Some patients are diagnosed solely on the basis of laboratory tests of the fluid bathing the brain and spinal cord and present no symptoms at all. Others have a dramatic variety, often occurring early in the history of the disease, called meningovascular syphilis, in which a sudden occlusion of a major blood vessel produces rapid death of some area of the brain or spinal cord, with symptoms and signs of loss of function in the specific dead area. Such patients may appear to have suffered an ordinary "stroke," for example, with weakness or paralysis of one side of the body.

The more characteristic varieties of neurosyphilis are paresis and tabes dorsalis. Both result from slowly progressive death of nerve cells. Paretics can show everything from minor personality changes to frank psychosis. Memory loss, euphoria, trouble in speaking, and delusions are common. Tabes dorsalis is caused by degeneration of the backmost section of the spinal cord, in which run certain sensory pathways from the limbs to the brain. Tabetics have an unsteady gait, a loss of reflexes, strange feelings in their extremities, impotency, trouble emptying their bladders, and sometimes "lightning pains," sudden agonizing shooting pains down their legs. Some of these patients have abdominal "crises" with vomiting and severe belly pain. Because of the diseased sensory pathways, damage to the joints may occur, and the patient may end up with a "bag of bones"—an abnormally mobile joint with severe destruction of the bony surfaces making up the joint.

The eyes may also be involved in late neurosyphilis. The optic nerve may atrophy, with constriction of the visual fields (so-called "tunnel vision"). The pupils may be small and irregular and do not respond normally to light. The normal pupil dilates in the dark and constricts when a light is shined into the eye; the syphilitic pupil responds only to changes in focusing for near or far objects.

Tertiary cardiovascular syphilis is caused by a degeneration of the middle layer of the aorta, the biggest artery in the body. As a result, the wall weakens. If it weakens in the area of the aortic valve, which is close to the heart, there is widening of the aortic ring and leaking of blood back into the heart after ejection of blood with each heart beat. Eventually this leads to heart failure. If the disease afflicts the area where the coronary arteries take off from the aorta, the patient may suffer from angina pectoris. If the weakness in the aorta occurs further along, there may be no symptoms unless the so-called "aneurysm" (a localized arterial outpouching or widening) begins to press on nearby structures. A big aortic aneurysm may cause hoarseness by pressure on the laryngeal nerve, or back pain by eroding the spine, or (rarely) may actually rupture through the chest wall. The manifestations of late syphilis remind one of the warning in Deuteronomy: "The Lord shall smite thee with madness, and blindness, and astonishment of heart."

The treponema of syphilis, unlike other nonviral microorganisms, has no difficulty crossing the placenta, so that the fetus residing in a syphilitic mother's uterus is an easy target for infection. When the mother is in the primary or secondary stages of syphilis, there is usually a massive invasion of the fetus by spirochetes, and the result is an abortion—after the fourth month, since the spirochetes cannot cross the placenta and infect the fetus before that—or a stillborn infant. If the mother has had syphilis for a long time, she may give birth to an uninfected child. Infection of the child can be prevented by adequate treatment of the mother before the eighteenth week of pregnancy. An already infected fetus can also be treated after this time, since antibiotics given to the mother will readily pass the placenta.

Early congenital syphilis is the term applied to those manifestations of syphilis that appear before the age of two years. Shortly after birth, a syphilitic baby may have small or large blisters, which become crusted sores; this is in contrast to acquired syphilis in adults, where blisters are never seen. Later on, skin lesions similar to those seen in adults appear.

The mucous membranes of the nose and pharynx are often involved, with the production of a heavy mucoid discharge referred to as "the snuffles." (A baby with a bloody nasal discharge almost always has syphilis.) The skin and the mucous membrane lesions are teeming with spirochetes, facilitating not only diagnosis by dark-field microscopy but also the spread of infection.

The skeleton is afflicted with an inflammation of the bone and cartilage. There is usually an anemia, and two-thirds of cases have a big liver and spleen, sometimes associated with mild jaundice.

If syphilis is untreated and persists after two years of age, the child enters the stage of late congenital syphilis. At this point the child is no longer infectious, and indeed may show nothing other than a positive blood test. Some infected children, however, may display one or more of the following disorders:

1. *Interstitial keratitis,* in which the cornea looks like ground glass. It is usually bilateral, appears around puberty, and may cause blindness.

2. *Hutchinson's teeth,* due to maldevelopment of the central incisors. These teeth are barrel- or screwdriver-shaped, notched, smaller than usual, and hence more widely spaced. X-rays of the mouth can diagnose this disease of the permanent teeth before they erupt.

3. *Mulberry molars,* a term applied to the deformed first molars, which show abnormal cusps that give the bottom of these teeth the look of a mulberry.

4. *Bone involvement,* which can take several forms. The shin bone can be thickened and bowed forward— the so-called "saber shin." The frontal bones (the forehead) can be thickened and "bossed." The nose or hard palate can be destroyed, leading to "saddle nose" or palatal perforation. Any part of the skeletal system may be involved.

5. *Skin lesions,* including gummas and cracks or fissures around the mouth or nose.

6. *Painless swelling of the joints* due to fluid accumulation. These swellings usually occur in the knees, less often in the elbows or other big joints.

7. *Central nervous system disease,* which can be like the paresis and tabes seen in adults or may take the form of deafness, often coming on at puberty but sometimes delayed until middle age.

8. *Cardiovascular lesions,* which are rarely seen.

Because the joint manifestations, keratitis, and deafness all come on around puberty, are commonly associated, respond poorly to penicillin or other antibiotics, and may respond to drugs of the cortisone group, these forms of congenital syphilis are thought by many to be, like gummas, hypersensitivity phenomena rather than direct results of spirochetal involvement.

We must now turn to gonorrhea. While syphilis can be a catastrophic disease in many ways, it is numerically far less important than gonorrhea, of which there are about twenty cases for every one of syphilis. Unlike syphilis, the time course of gonococcal disease is rapid. Its causative organism is *Neisseria gonorrhoeae*, a diplococcal bacterium consisting of two kidney- or bean-shaped organisms.

As with most venereal diseases, the medical profession has derided the concept that gonorrhea could be acquired by nonvenereal contact. But a disquieting minority view about the old toilet-seat theory was voiced in 1973 by a Swedish physician named Claes Henning. He smeared a suspension of gonococci on various surfaces in a washroom and then tried to reisolate the bugs. Even after four hours he succeeded in growing some from a washbasin, a water tap, an electric light switch, a damp cotton towel, and—hold your breath—a toilet seat. In some cases they were still present twenty-four hours later, although the numbers decreased enormously even in the first few hours. What these experiments mean is not entirely clear, but Dr. Henning suggests that dirty restrooms can be a menace and that the patient who denies that sexual contact is the cause of his gonorrhea may be telling the truth (20). One suspects that the Swedish doctor may be right in theory, but that in practice the toilet seat is usually an innocent by-sitter. On the other hand, two other Swedish scientists have grown gonococci from towels soiled by urethral discharge from infected males (21). Some bacteria were still alive twenty-four hours later.

In men, the diagnosis is relatively easy. Within one to fourteen days after sexual exposure to an infected partner, the patient develops painful urination and a penile discharge of yellow, creamy pus in which one can find the causative organism. If untreated, the infection may invade the prostate or the epididymis, which lies alongside the testis. In many infected females, although the cervix, vagina, and urethra are affected, there may be no symptoms and the discharge may not attract attention. Some women, however, will complain of a yellow vaginal discharge and experience frequency of urination, painful urination, occasionally bloody urine, backache, abdominal discomfort prior to the menstrual period, or heavy menstrual flow. If untreated, the gonococcus can cause inflammation and abscess formation in the fallopian tubes or ovaries, with the possibility of permanent infertility.

The gonococcus does not necessarily confine its mischief to the genitourinary tract. It may invade the blood stream and seed itself on the valves of the heart or the brain coverings (with resultant meningitis) (22), or in various joints, or in the eye. The latter site is particularly at risk in the baby born of an infected mother; such infants can develop blindness if the infection is severe. (It is to prevent gonococcal eye inflammation that silver nitrate or penicillin drops are routinely put into the eyes of newborns; unfortunately the prophylactic procedures sometimes fail [23, 24].) Infection to the infant is transmitted by direct contact between the baby and the infected tissues of the mother; unlike syphilis, gonorrhea cannot spread from the blood stream of the mother into the infant because the gonococcus cannot cross the placenta.

While some of these gonococcal migrations can be associated with dramatic disease, it is now recognized that the spread of the organism can also produce a relatively mild form of disease which is especially hard to diagnose. This occurs more often in women, because they are less likely to receive prompt diagnosis and treatment. The picture is a triad of fever, arthritis, and skin lesions. The fever is usually moderate and may begin with a shaking chill. The joints affected are usually those in the limbs and can be either small or large ones. Some have fluid in them, others do not. The rashes are of several kinds: raised lesions, pimples, blisters, or hives. The disease is easy to confuse with such nonvenereal diseases as rheumatic fever, rheumatoid arthritis, drug reactions, and serum sickness.

In recent years, gonococcal infections of the pharynx and rectum have come in for greater attention than previously. Women who practice fellatio can contract pharyngeal and tonsillar gonococcal disease; oral and rectal gonorrhea seem to be special problems in male homosexuals. Symptoms of rectal gonorrhea can be absent (the majority of patients are asymptomatic) or extremely annoying. Rectal itching, pain, or burning may be accompanied by a bloody or mucoid discharge. Diarrhea is rare. The symptoms of gonococcal pharyngitis or tonsillitis are no different from what one would see in an ordinary throat infection, such as a streptococcal sore throat. The patient, one or two days after exposure, complains of throat pain and perhaps shows a little fever or enlarged lymph glands in the neck.

Gonorrhea cannot be spread by kissing, and it is believed that the patient with gonococcal pharyngitis cannot spread infection to a partner by performing cunnilingus. The reason for this is that the oral mucosa resembles skin more than it does other mucous membranes and is resistant to the gonococcus. The saliva also exerts an antibacterial action, so that it is really in the lymphoid tissue of the tonsils that the gonococcus can set up shop. The reverse is not true, however—a patient with gonococcal vaginitis or urethritis can certainly infect a partner who performs orogenital contact.

There are a number of other venereal diseases, but they are much less common. Chancroid, caused by the Ducrey bacillus, causes painful multiple ulcers on the penis or vulva. Lymphogranuloma venereum is due to a small viruslike organism of the Bedsonia group. The primary genital lesion is small and transient. Some weeks later the glands in the groin are affected, as well as some in the abdomen (the latter may mimic acute appendicitis). The groin lesions can break down; they may lead to such extensive scar tissue that serious swelling of the genitals can ensue. Infection can spread to the rectum and there cause ulceration and eventually scarring.

Granuloma inguinale is a rare condition caused by the "Donovan body," a bacterium. Lesions appear on the groin and the genitals and develop into raised, red, velvety surfaces that bleed easily. They may turn into cancer, which probably explains why cancer of the vulva and penis are both frequently seen in young people in Jamaica, where granuloma inguinale is not uncommon.

There are other diseases which are not often thought of as venereal but are transmitted by sexual contact. One is trichomoniasis, which produces a yellow, frothy vaginal discharge. Another is moniliasis, caused by a yeast, *Candida albicans*, and manifested by a white vaginal discharge and itchiness of the anal and groin areas. The skin of the genitalia, thighs, and perineum may be red, shiny, and fissured, and white patches can be seen on the vulvar or penile mucosa. Scabies and lice can also be transmitted by close contact.

A disease that seems to be growing in importance is nongonococcal urethritis. In the De Kalb County, Georgia, VD clinic, it is as prevalent as gonorrhea (25), and at the University of Virginia it is actually much more common than gonorrhea (26). The ailment afflicts middle-class white men more often than it does lower-class blacks. The urethral exudate is typically scant and clear, as opposed to the profuse, purulent discharge of gonorrhea; both are associated with burning and pain on urination. The etiology of the disease is uncertain: some suspect so-called "T-strain" mycoplasmas; others implicate *Chlamydia trachomatis,* which also causes conjunctivitis in both children and adults (27, 28). Nongonococcal urethritis, unlike gonorrhea, does not respond to penicillin, but may to tetracycline. Treatment failures and relapses are not uncommon.

It is traditional to restrict the term "venereal" to those ailments that are almost never spread *except* by sexual contact. However, reports continue to appear implicating a venereal mode of spread for diseases generally not considered sex-related. Two of the latest are viral hepatitis, which has been found in several studies to occur with greater than expected frequency in sexually promiscuous people (especially prostitutes [29] and homosexuals [30, 31]), and histoplasmosis. The latter is due to a fungus and usually resembles tuberculosis, but a recent paper described penile and vulvar lesions in a man and wife.

There is a school of thought that believes that cervical cancer may be venereal (32). A herpes virus—related to the one that causes "cold sores"—has been incriminated. Infection of the genitalia with herpes virus occurs in 1 in 3,000 women in higher socioeconomic groups, but in 1 in 250 women in lower socieconomic strata. Three out of four women who have sexual contact with infected men will develop a herpes infection. Studies at Johns Hopkins suggest that 98 percent of women with cancerous or precancerous changes in the cervix have once been infected with herpes virus. The theory is that the virus lies dormant until certain stresses (such as hormonal changes) activate it, thus leading to cancer. It has been known for a long time that cervical cancer is extremely rare in virgins and most common in prostitutes or sexually promiscuous women. There is, sad to say, no way at present to eradicate this virus, which is causing venereal infections at a rate which is reported to be dramatically increasing.

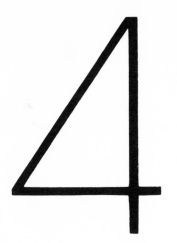

VD
in the
Laboratory

For most of recorded history, the venereal diseases have been studied as clinical phenomena, not as reasons for laboratory study. This is a characteristic of all diseases, since medicine is old and science is relatively young. For the last century, however, VD has invaded the laboratories of microbiologists and immunologists, as scientists searched both for a better understanding of these important ailments and for better ways of diagnosing their presence.

The simplest and quickest way to diagnose syphilis is to see the causative corkscrew in material scraped from a chancre or secondary lesions. This is done by "darkfield microscopy," which is so called because the specimen is not brilliantly illuminated (as would be the case for most things a microscopist would look at), but is faintly illuminated from the sides. This procedure is used because the spirochete is so thin that ordinary light microscopy doesn't provide enough power of resolution. The syphilis-causing spirochete, *Treponema pallidum,* is easy to tell from most other spirochetes when it is in motion but not after it has been dried and stained, the traditional way of examining most microorganisms.

In performing a darkfield examination, the physician or technician must wear plastic or rubber gloves as protection against accidental infection. The suspected lesion is cleaned with saline solution, dried, and gently abraded to the point of bleeding. The lesion is then pressed until clear serum exudes. A drop of this serum is placed on a glass slide and a thin coverslip placed over it. If there is to be any delay in examination, the edges are sealed with jelly to prevent the specimen's drying out. A darkfield condenser is used to block out the central rays of light and direct the peripheral rays from the side onto the material under study. One can only see those rays that are reflected up into the eyepiece by an object on the slide, which then looks light against a dark background, the way dust in the air is made visible when a ray of sunlight enters a dark room.

Treponema pallidum, the cause of syphilis, moves slowly forward and backward, rotating around its long axis like a corkscrew, with slight bending and twisting from side to side. In motion, another spirochete, *T. refringens,* is less delicate than *T. pallidum*—its spirals are less rigid and their conformation changes greatly as the treponeme swims. There is an innocent relative, *T. microdentium,* which does not cause disease but looks almost identical to *T. pallidum.* Fortunately for the diagnostician, *T. microdentium* is only found in the mouth, at the margins of the gums or beneath the gums. Lesions on the lips, the inside of the mouth, the tongue, or the throat from which a spirochete that looks like *T. pallidum* is isolated can be assumed to be syphilitic; only when a chancre or secondary lesion is present on the gums is it hard to know how to interpret the presence of spirochetes.

The syphilis spirochete dies quickly outside the body and is readily killed by drying or by exposure to soap and water. By contrast, motile spirochetes have been found in infected cadavers kept in a mortuary for forty-eight hours. Indeed, one can freeze spirochetes at $-70°C$ and infect an animal with the thawed organisms nine years later.

The isolation of suspicious-looking spirochetes, while quick and definitive, is less useful generally as a diagnostic and epidemiologic aid than is the blood test. Current theory holds that when *T. pallidum* invades a human host, it acts as an antigen (a stimulator of antibody formation) and evokes the production of multiple antibodies of two basic types—nonspecific and specific. The nonspecific antibodies are called reagins and underlie the Wassermann test (see below). Reagins are directed against a fatty antigen of the spirochete, or against a fatty antigen that results when spirochete and host interact. Since antigens of this kind occur in normal tissues, tests based on them can be "falsely positive" when a patient does not have syphilis, a cause of distress to doctor and patient that will be discussed shortly.

The specific antitreponemal antibodies use some preparation of the treponema itself as the antigen, so that a positive test of this type is usually quite specific. It does not, however, necessarily mean an active infection, since antibodies may persist long after an infection.

The first blood test for syphilis dates back to 1906 and is named after August von Wassermann, who was director of the Institute for Experimental Therapy in Dahlem, a suburb of Berlin. Wassermann stumbled upon his antigen by a happy stroke of luck. Looking for a rich source of spirochetes to serve as a specific antigen, he made an extract of fetal liver from a case of congenital syphilis. The lucky break lay in the fact that a substance in normal tissues reacted with syphilitic sera in the test tube exactly like the extract of syphilitic liver. While Wassermann suspected that normal tissue might well be less specific than infected tissue, he was willing to settle for a certain degree of nonspecificity in view of the greater convenience.

The nonspecific tests most commonly employed today are the Venereal Disease Research Laboratory (VDRL) and the Kolmer tests. At one time, several such tests were often run simultaneously, but now most authorities recommend picking one of these and concentrating on making it reproducible. Why, you may ask, does anyone want to use a *nonspecific* test? The reasons are simple: these tests are easy to run, cheap, and can be quantitated. None of these is true for the specific tests.

Most laboratories report the result as the highest dilution (titer) of the patient's serum that still gives a positive test (1:64, for example). Such titers are sometimes helpful in diagnosis, but are particularly useful in following the response of a patient to therapy. Titers may range from zero to high in primary syphilis, are commonly high (1:1024 or higher can be seen) in secondary syphilis, and variable in later stages. False-positive reactors usually do not have titers above 1:8. Sometimes the antibody titer is so high in secondary syphilis that undiluted serum for some reason gives a negative test; only on dilution does it become positive. Since perhaps 1 percent of secondary syphilitics show this "prozone phenomenon," it is a pity that many laboratories do not test the patient's diluted serum unless the undiluted serum is positive.

The first specific treponemal test was the TPI or treponemal immobilization test, which was devised in 1949 by Nelson and Mayer. These investigators used virulent *Treponema pallidum* extracted from the testicles of infected rabbits and placed them in media known to allow their survival for at least brief periods of time. Serum from a patient was then added, along with complement (a plasma factor needed to make many antigen-antibody reactions "go") from normal serum. They then counted the percentage of spirochetes that were immobilized and compared this with control serum.

The test was ingenious and rightfully earned great kudos for its inventors, even though two-thirds of patients with primary syphilis and one-third with secondary syphilis were judged negative by it, and it was positive in patients infected by treponemes other than the one causing syphilis. With the passage of time, however, disenchantment set in. In theory simple, the test proved a nightmare in practice. Each laboratory needed a colony of rabbits as well as highly trained and skilled technicians. The results varied enormously from one lab to another, and it was found that the results were critically dependent on the media used, the amount of added complement, the incubation time, the number of spirochetes counted, and whether the infected rabbits were pretreated with cortisonelike drugs or x-ray. The presence of antibiotics in the serum invalidates the test, since antibiotics will inactivate motile treponemes.

Later substitutes fared no better until the application of immunofluorescent methods, which have revolutionized diagnostic microbiology. The principle here is simple: the bug (or its antigen) is mixed with the patient's serum. Antibodies to the bug latch onto the antigen, and the whole complex is then made visible by adding an antibody *to the antibody* (antihuman gamma globulin), which is labeled with a fluorescent material readily seen by appropriate microscopic inspection.

The test of this sort used today is the fluorescent treponemal antibody absorption test (FTA-ABS). The original version was very sensitive in all stages of syphilis but was often positive in uninfected people. These false positives could be eliminated by diluting the patient's serum 1:200 before the test, but then the test missed detecting people who were known to be syphilitic. The present version treats a 1:5 dilution of the patient's serum with an extract of a culture of a non-pathogenic treponeme, which removes an antibody common to all sorts of treponemes, including those that live saprophytically in man without causing infection. As now performed in most state health laboratories, the FTA-ABS test is positive in 95 to 99 percent of cases of secondary, late, or latent syphilis, 85 percent of primary syphilis, and "falsely" positive in only a very few patients, most of whom have diseases associated with abnormal globulin proteins in their sera. By contrast, the VDRL is positive in only 75 percent or so of all types except the secondary phase, where its batting average is about as high as the FTA-ABS. The TPI (when performed properly) is about as good as the FTA-ABS in all except the primary cases, when it misses almost 50 percent of infections.

An interesting survey, which gives insight into the validity of both the FTA-ABS and the VDRL tests, was performed in a population of nuns (33). A total of 250 nuns volunteered for the study. All the participants denied sexual contact or a history of congenital or acquired syphilis. None of the bloods tested were positive by the VDRL test, but three were positive by the FTA-ABS test. Two of these three women were over fifty years of age and had a history or abnormalities in physical examination compatible with rheumatoid arthritis. The third reactor was also positive by TPI test. Since she had spent a year in Peru about forty years prior to the experiment, it is conceivable that she had suffered a mild infection of pinta or yaws, treponemal infections common in that part of the world.

It is necessary to do the FTA-ABS test in any patient

suspected of having latent syphilis of the central nervous or cardiovascular systems, since the VDRL test is falsely negative in as many as a third of such cases. On the other hand, the tendency of the FTA-ABS to stay positive forever makes the VDRL the best test for following response to treatment.

There is a special problem of diagnosis in newborn infants who show positive tests but who are clinically normal. (The child with the clear-cut signs of syphilis described in Chapter 3 poses no difficulties.) Has such a child been infected or has there merely occurred a passive transfer of maternal antibody? If the latter is the case, the infant's VDRL titer is usually not greater than that of the mother's serum and usually declines sharply in the first two or three months of life. It is not an appealing set of options for the doctor, however; he has no desire either to delay treatment of a truly infected infant or to treat needlessly a nonsyphilitic baby. There has, therefore, been considerable interest in developing a sensitive and specific test for congenital syphilis. Thus far the best seems to be a fluorescein-labeled antibody against one of the major types of human immune globulin in a modified FTA-ABS; early reports are promising.

The situation with regard to congenital syphilis is made even nastier by the fact that a mother who acquires syphilis late in pregnancy may give birth to a child with a negative blood test. Such children, apparently normal at birth, may develop clinical syphilis one to many months later.

It is always disturbing to have the lab report a positive VDRL blood test for syphilis on a patient with no stigmata or history of syphilis. One possibility is a laboratory error, so the test should be promptly repeated. If it comes back positive a second time, and the titer has not changed and no signs of syphilis have appeared, the patient either has latent syphilis or a false positive test. The next step is to do a more specific test, such as the FTA-ABS. If the latter is negative, the patient probably has a false positive reaction to the VDRL.

Such false positive reactions are, unfortunately, not uncommon. The percentage in various series involving the VDRL test has run from 3 to 40 percent (34). In one large Massachusetts survey, 3 percent of nonwhite patients and 28 percent of whites had apparent false positives; the figure for clinic patients was 15 percent as opposed to 30 percent of private patients. Boston, the largest city in the state, had the lowest overall percentage of false positives. There is thus a distinct socioeconomic correlation.

Some false positive reactors revert to normal (in the absence of treatment) in less than six months. Most of these instances occur after various immunizations or nonsyphilitic infections such as measles, tuberculosis, chicken pox, scarlet fever, leprosy, or pneumonia. The chronic false positive reactor, on the other hand, often has a serious or chronic underlying disease such as lupus erythematosus, thyroiditis, rheumatoid arthritis, or cancer. Occasionally, a drug-induced sensitivity state can be at fault.

For reasons that are obscure, heroin addicts and the aged are also likely to show false positive reactions. For narcotic addicts the figure is very high—about 20 to 25 percent, and these reactions may persist for as long as a year after the patient is off illicit drugs. The incidence of false positives also increases with age. Whereas only 1.7 percent of 10,000 men aged fifty-five to sixty had a false positive VDRL test in one large study, a 9 to 10 percent rate has been reported in patients seventy to eighty years old (35, 36, 37). These elderly patients generally have low titers and an increase in the serum concentrations of such things as total globulins and the so-called rheumatoid factor. The meaning of such tests in the aged is unclear, except that knowledge of the phenomenon is important if aged patients are not to be needlessly alarmed or treated.

The success of scientists in devising blood tests for syphilis contrasts vividly with their failure to do the same for gonorrhea. In a sense, to be sure, the development of sensitive selective media by Thayer and Martin in 1964 has so facilitated the isolation of the gonococcus in the bacteriological laboratory that there has been less incentive for devising workable serological tests. Nevertheless, since infected women are frequently unaware of gonococcal infection, case finding on a mass scale would be greatly facilitated—and indeed perhaps only make sense—if a blood test for gonorrhea were available. There is an old test, called "complement fixation," which tests for antibodies in the blood against a suspension of gonococci. It is rarely positive in uninfected patients, but may miss the presence of infection in anywhere from 30 to 80 percent of people with active gonorrhea—hardly an admirable performance.

Attempts have been made using the antigen from gonococci treated in different ways (ultrasonic disintegration, for example), but the results were only slightly more encouraging than with the older test. Research in this problem would probably be facilitated by definitive information on the exact antigenic structure of the gonococcus and of possible differences between the various strains of this bug. A few years ago, for example, a virulent new strain of gonococcus appeared in California. The disease it caused was called Asian or Vietnamese gonorrhea, since it was believed by some to have been introduced into the United States by military personnel returning from Southeast Asia. (Others believed it to be the result of natural mutations.)

New York State Health Department scientists have been working with a blood test that causes fluorescence of heat-stable gonococcal antibodies under an ultraviolet microscope, but further experience is required before it is known how useful this test will prove to be. Its current status is described further in Chapter 8.

The laboratory has also been the site of numerous attempts to produce venereal disease in animals. A successful animal model for gonorrhea has been sought since early in the nineteenth century. In 1948, Miller inoculated the anterior chamber of a rabbit's eye with the gonococcus and produced an experimental infection in the eye. In 1971, three scientists from the Public Health Service VD Research Laboratory in Atlanta transferred gonorrhea to the urethras of three male chimpanzees (38). The chimps all developed typical gonorrheal urethritis. (One chimp even gave himself gonococcal conjunctivitis, presumably by manual transfer.) The infection was also subsequently transmitted from chimpanzee to chimpanzee. Nor did the USPHS scientists stop there. They paired some infected male chimps with a healthy female chimp. The lady chimp came down with a mild form of infection, similar to the "silent" infection so often found in human females. It thus appears that an animal model for human gonorrhea finally had been found. Such a model should prove helpful in blood testing research, as well as in the study of vaccines or drug therapy.

Treponemes, too, have been extensively studied in the laboratory. Over seventy strains have been isolated, most from humans, a few from rabbits. About half of the human strains were isolated from syphilitics, the others from patients suffering from related diseases such as yaws.

The hamster is the best laboratory animal for isolating treponemes. After isolation, the spirochetes are transferred to rabbits, by inoculating either into the testicles or onto the skin of the back or scrotum. After a lag of a day or two, the treponemes begin to multiply logarithmically. (It is estimated that it takes about thirty hours for a spirochete to divide.) About a hundred million spirochetes are required to produce a lesion visible to the naked eye. One can produce small local lesions in monkeys with rabbit strains of treponeme, but such spirochetes rarely produce generalized disease in this species.

A number of variables are known to affect the course of laboratory infection. If one raises the environmental temperature above 35°C (95°F), the bugs have a hard time living, and at 40°C (104°F) there is progressive destruction of the treponemes. Below 30°C, they probably don't multiply, either. Since the rabbit's natural body temperature is 39°C (higher than the 37° or so that is normal for man), it is probably not surprising that one rarely sees syphilitic lesions of the rabbit's internal organs. A rabbit's skin, ears, testicles, and extremities, however, are cooler, and those are the places where the treponemes grow. (At one time, human syphilis was actually treated by injecting microorganisms or other foreign protein to produce fever.)

One can only speculate as to what this relationship to ambient temperature may mean for human infection. In the tropics, skin temperature is slightly but definitely higher than in more temperate climes. Has this had an adverse effect on the spirochete of syphilis? Has it made it less virulent over the years? Has the higher temperature made the spirochete less antigenic, leading in turn to poor development of immune responses and hence a tendency for the disease to have a more chronic course, with relapses over a period of years?

We do know that certain diseases exist in the tropics that are caused by spirochetes that look exactly like *T.*

pallidum under the microscope. Two of these diseases are pinta and yaws, and the causative organisms are called, respectively, *Treponema carateum* and *Treponema pertenue*, but the only way to "identify" them is to know the nature of the disease they cause. Pinta means "painted" and refers to the typical change in pigmentation of the skin seen in this disease. Yaws patients have characteristic mulberry-shaped skin sores, which explains why the disease is also called frambesia (from the French *framboise* for raspberry). Both diseases usually start in children, but are never congenital. The diseases spread by skin contact, and the patients are infectious for years. Both ailments affect the skin first. Yaws can afflict bones; pinta does not. No other organs are involved in either disease. Blood tests for syphilis are also positive in these ailments, and the diseases respond well to antibiotics.

Hormones, too, can alter the response of animals to treponemal infections. Male rabbits, for example, get a worse disease than do female rabbits. Cortisone treatment, by suppressing inflammatory and antibody response, allows the spirochetes to overgrow fantastically. After sudden withdrawal of the cortisone, things get even worse. There is a tremendous increase in the size of the lesions, often with the development of extensive generalized lesions.

Antibiotics, not surprisingly, interfere with the production of experimental infections in animals. Disaster has occasionally struck a laboratory working on treponemal infections as the result of unknown antibiotic contamination of the feed for the animals by a well-intentioned supplier.

Immunity to treponemes develops slowly in infected laboratory animals, over weeks and months. Its development and persistence depends on such variables as how extensive the infection is, how long it has lasted, and when the animal is rechallenged with new spirochetes. One interesting (and perhaps depressing) bit of information is the fact that an animal can be resistant to local reinfection while harboring virulent spirochetes in its lymph nodes.

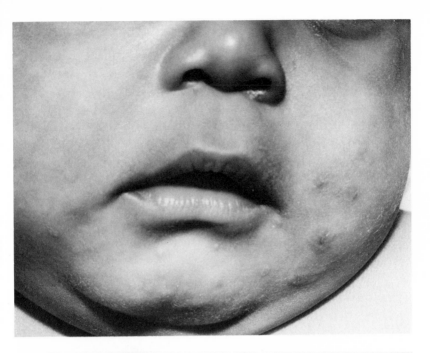

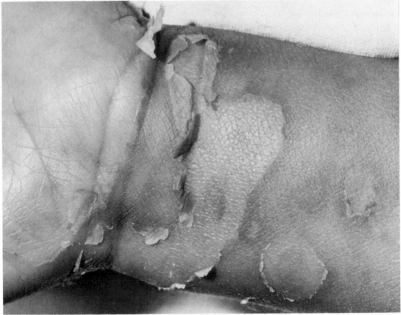

Congenital syphilis in a 3½-month-old child—facial rash and skin lesions (courtesy of the Skin and Cancer Hospital, Temple University)

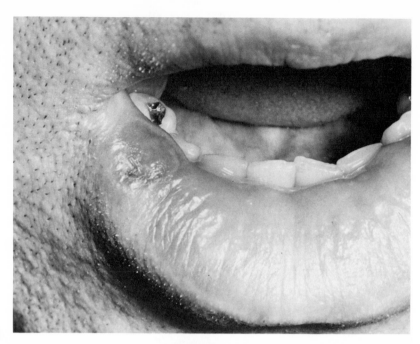

Primary syphilis—
chancres of the lip and
penis (courtesy of the
Skin and Cancer
Hospital, Temple
University)

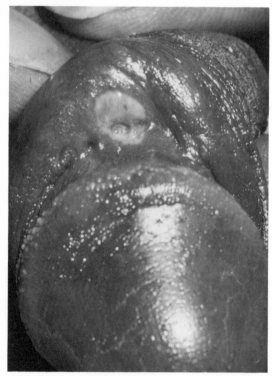

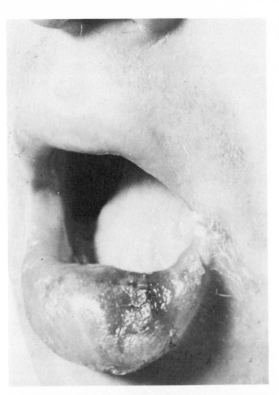

Secondary syphilis—
healing primary chancres
of the lip and penis
(courtesy of the Skin and
Cancer Hospital, Temple
University)

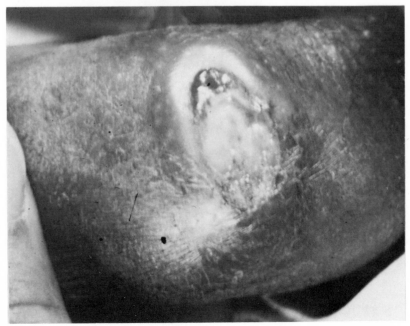

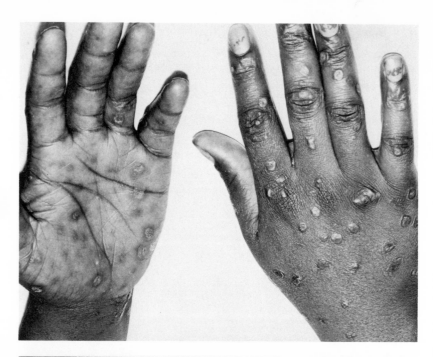

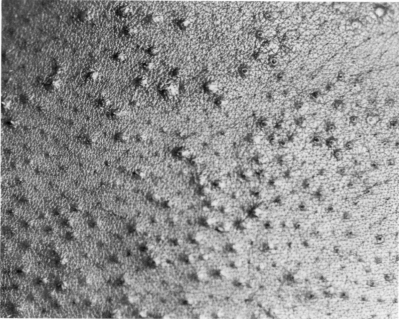

Secondary syphilis—two types of rash (courtesy of the Skin and Cancer Hospital, Temple University)

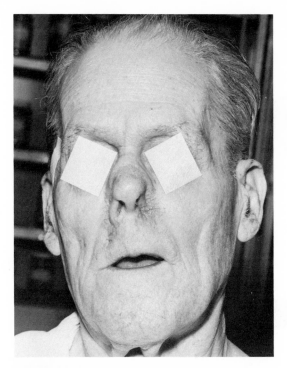

Tertiary syphilis—
examples of saddle nose
(courtesy of the Skin and
Cancer Hospital, Temple
University)

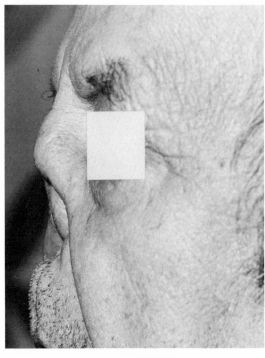

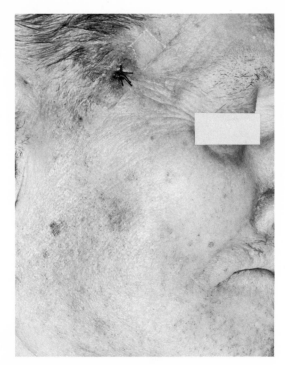

Tertiary syphilis—skin
manifestations and
perforated palate
(courtesy of the Skin and
Cancer Hospital, Temple
University)

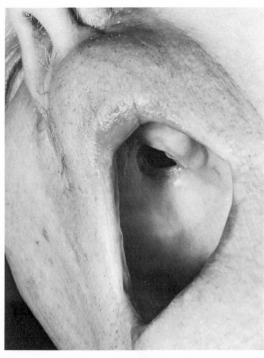

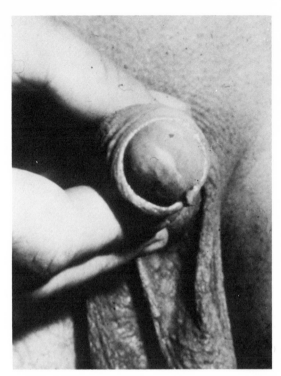

Gonorrhea—characteristic penile discharge as it appears to the eye and under the microscope in a stained smear showing the gonococcus, *Neisseria gonorrhoeae* (courtesy of the Center for Disease Control, U.S. Public Health Service)

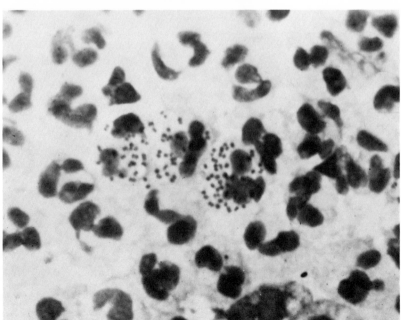

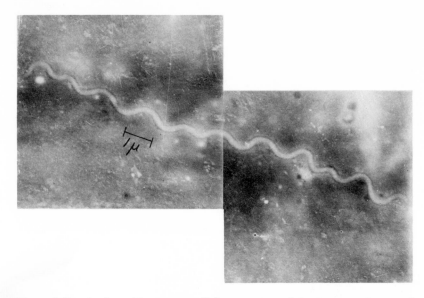

The syphilis spirochete, *Treponema pallidum* (courtesy of the American Society of Microbiology)

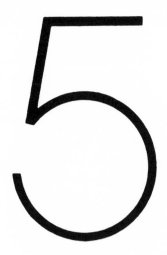

Heavy Metals and the Tuskegee Scandal

In 1812, William Fergusson, Inspector General of Hospitals to the Portuguese Army, wrote the following:

> Syphilis has excited much interest and attention in this country on the part of all British medical observers; no less from its dreadful ravages amongst their own countrymen, than from its comparatively milder phaenomena amongst the inhabitants of the country. In the British army, . . . venereal ulceration has not only been more intractable to the operation of mercury than under similar circumstances at home, but the constitution, while strongly under the influence of the remedy, has become affected with the secondary symptoms in a proportion that could not have been expected. With the natives, on the contrary, the disease is very mild; curable, for the most part, by topical treatment alone, or wearing itself out, when received into the constitution, after running a certain course (not always a very destructive one) without the use of any adequate mercurial remedy. . . . I have lived long enough amongst them to ascertain, that their return to hospital under such circumstances for secondary symptoms, is far from universal, or even a frequent occurrence (39).

Here was a "remedy" over three hundred years old, the most popular treatment for syphilis, that made the British troops who were treated with it worse off than the Portuguese soldiers whose syphilis went untreated. In fact, up until the middle of the nineteenth century, it was not clear which of the symptoms of treated patients were due to syphilis and which to mercury intoxication. Why was there so much confusion about the merits of this remedy?

The origins of mercury treatment for syphilis are nebulous. As early as 1615, Miguel Cervantes wrote satirically in his *Don Quixote:* "Virgilius forgot to tell us who was the first man in the world to have a cold in the head, or the first to take inunctions for the French disease" (40). We do know, however, that during the eleventh to thirteenth centuries many crusaders returned to Europe with what was called leprosy; some of them were treated with the mercury-containing Saracen's Ointment. But mercury ointment is effective in the treatment of a variety of skin disorders, especially those caused by parasites, so the popularity of this remedy neither proves that this "leprosy" was in fact syphilis nor that syphilis was curable by mercury.

Somewhere around the end of the fifteenth century —the exact date of publication is unknown—appeared the first known printed work in which mercury is mentioned as a possible cure for syphilis. The author was Konrad Schellig, a Heidelberg professor and personal physician to Count-Palatinate Philip. At least seven other European authors advised such treatment around the same time.

Pedro Pintor (1423–1503) practiced medicine in Rome and treated some famous people with mercury, including the Borgia pope, Alexander VI, and other members of the Borgia family. The results were not always happy, but his lack of success with these distinguished personages and the Cardinal of Segovia did not prevent any number of high-ranking churchmen from seeking his dubious treatment.

Giovanni de Vigo, a contemporary physician, decided to improve on the standard mercury preparations by putting live frogs in with quicksilver in the preparation of his ointment.

Fracastorius, the man who gave the world the term "syphilis" in his long poem *Syphilidis sive de Morbo Gallico*, ("Syphilis or the French Disease"), was a respected physician. His famous work included his therapeutic views on the treatment of syphilis, despite the fact that these views met with the disfavor of his patron, Cardinal Pietro Bembo, who preferred that syphilis be treated with guaiac, also known as lignum sanctum, or Holy Wood. Fracastorius describes the introduction of mercury with the story of Ilceus, who was struck by syphilis as punishment for killing a deer sacred to Diana and was then allegedly cured by bathing three times in a stream of quicksilver, the healing fluid being poured over him by a custodian nymph. In the allegory, Fracastorius demonstrates a certain ambivalence toward the treatment, saying at one point that treating the entire body with mercury might cause choking and difficult breathing, but in another section pointing out that "most people do better by dissolving everything in quicksilver, since the power inherent in this is wonderful" (40).

Benvenuto Cellini, in his *Autobiography*, boasts of having been a victim of syphilis:

> It was true, indeed, that I had got the sickness; but I believe I caught it from that fine young servant girl whom I was keeping when my house was robbed. The French disease, for it was that, remained in me dormant before it showed itself, and then it broke out

over my whole body at one instant. It was not like what one commonly observes, but covered my flesh with certain blisters, of the size of six pences, and rose colored. The doctors would not call it the French disease, albeit I told them why I thought it was that. I went on treatment myself according with their methods, but derived no benefit (41, 42).

Later, when his life was plotted against, Cellini was fed large doses of calomel (mercurous chloride). He planned legal recourse against his enemies and called in physicians and surgeons because he feared that the mercury had "corroded my intestines." Upon recovering, however, he not only felt well but also believed himself cured of his syphilis. At this point, he honored his would-be murderers as therapists, saying, "God sent us evil that it may work us good" (41, 42).

Nonetheless, Cellini has some caustic comments to make about a client-physician of his who became famous because of his mercury therapy:

> There arrived in Rome a surgeon of the highest renown, who was called Maestro Giacomo da Carpi. This able man, in the course of his practice, undertook the most desperate cases of the so-called French disease. In Rome this kind of illness is very partial to the priests, and especially to the richest of them. When, therefore, Maestro Giacomo had made his talents known, he professed to work miracles in the treatment of such cases by means of certain fumigations; but he only undertook a cure after stipulating his fees, which he reckoned not by tens, but by hundreds of crowns (40).

A later commentator, Fallopius, also spoke disparagingly of Carpi as a doctor more wealthy than skilled. Fallopius asserts that in the process of becoming rich through his treatment of the French disease, Carpi killed a great many patients with mercury inunctions.

In the sixteenth century the use of mercury proved even more profitable to the barber-surgeons, the alchemists, and the charlatans. Indeed, it has been said that syphilis was what finally allowed the alchemists to turn mercury into gold. There is a story about a barber-surgeon who was seen praying at the statue of Charles VIII in Paris. Upbraided because the statue was not that of a saint, the surgeon retorted that he knew what he was doing: "This man has given me an income of 7,000 lires" (40). The explanation is that syphilis was thought to have been spread through Europe by the soldiers in Charles's army and by their camp followers after an invasion of Italy in the late fifteenth century.

Paracelsus, the famous sixteenth-century figure who was part charlatan and part genius, was another powerful advocate of mercury. He vigorously attacked the "impostors" who used the Holy Wood in no less than nine books on the French Disease, and some historians believe that he was the first to prescribe mercury internally in the treatment of syphilis. Paracelsus did, however, also criticize those who used mercury in excess.

Not a man to mince words, Paracelsus made many enemies, and his books were suppressed. It has been suggested that the Fugger banking house was influential in this censorship because of a need to protect the revenue from their monopoly on the importation of Holy Wood from the New World, but the crafty Fuggers were also covering their bets by being deeply involved in the production of quicksilver.

Unlike Paracelsus, the French physician Jean Fernel refused to treat Francis I with mercury, and the king succumbed to syphilis. Fernel was more impressed with the toxic properties of mercury than with its therapeutic benefits, a posture which was definitely a minority opinion, but which was apparently shared by

Rabelais, the physician-author of *Gargantua and Pantagruel.* Rabelais gives an excellent clinical description of the toxic effects of mercury:

> But what shall I say of those poor men that are plagued with the pox and the gout? O how often have we seen them, even immediately after they are anointed and thoroughly greased, till their faces glister like the key-hole of a powdering tub, their teeth dance like the jacks of a little pair of organs or virginals, when they are played upon, and that they foamed with their very throats like a boar, which the mongrel mastiff-hounds have driven in (40).

The powdering tub that Rabelais mentions was a large wooden vat which could be used equally well to salt meat or to sweat and fumigate a syphilitic patient. Such tubs are also mentioned by Shakespeare and remained in use until the end of the nineteenth century.

It was not just patients who suffered from the treatments. Bernardino Ramazzini, the father of occupational medicine, describes the ill effects on surgeons of giving their patients mercury ointments:

> These persons belong to the lowest class of surgeons who carry on the business for the money to be made, for the better sort of surgeons avoid a service so disagreeable and a task so full of danger and hazard. Though they wear a glove when so engaged, it is impossible for them to prevent the mercurial atoms from penetrating the leather and so reaching the hand of him who applies the ointment; in fact, for other purposes, it is leather that we use for straining and clarifying mercury. For those who rub in this ointment I can suggest no sounder precautions than that employed by a surgeon of our day who had learned, to his cost, that his fee did not compensate for his own loss, since he found that the process of anointing did more harm to him than to those he

treated; for he was terribly afflicted by diarrhea, colic, and profuse salivation. So he now prepares the mercurial ointment and stays by the patients who are to be treated, but he orders them to rub in the ointment themselves with their own hand and declares this is better for him and for them (43).

Mercury continued to receive considerable attention in the medical literature down into our own century. The eighteenth century saw almost four hundred articles on the use of mercury in syphilis, and the next century about a thousand, with close to four hundred reports of intoxication from its use. In 1826 appeared the first paper on the subcutaneous injection of mercury, and the nineteenth century saw an impressive proliferation of different compounds of mercury for use by mouth, by application to the skin, or by injection. The metal did not actually disappear from medical use as an antisyphilitic until the advent of penicillin in the 1940's.

Goldwater has said, "The use of mercury in the treatment of syphilis may have been the most colossal hoax ever perpetrated in the history of a profession which has never been free of hoaxes" (40). The evidence in favor of mercury was both simple and simple-minded: persons thought to have syphilis and treated with mercury sometimes recovered. Yet we now know that the primary and secondary lesions of syphilis clear up spontaneously, often within a few weeks. We also know that, until the treponeme of syphilis was identified and the Wasserman test developed, the diagnosis of syphilis was often difficult and at times impossible.

In 1801, a critical physician named Tongue asked a provocative question in his M.D. dissertation for the University of Pennsylvania: "I should ask why, after having destroyed the venereal virus at its source; after having cured the original venereal ulcers, we should still see syphilitic affections in other parts of the body?" (44). Dr. Tongue had reason to be perplexed. Since the disappearance of local lesions under mercury ointment treatment was considered evidence of cure, why was not the appearance of new lesions evidence of failure? The patients of the world would have been spared a great deal of doctor-induced mercurial toxicity if this question had been answered centuries ago.

Mercury was only the first of the "heavy metals" to be used in the treatment of syphilis. The great Paul Ehrlich and a Japanese colleague named Sahachiro Hata, using rabbit syphilis as a test model, tested a long series of compounds, finally coming up, in 1909, with Salvarsan, the six-hundred-and-sixth compound examined. This "606," the Magic Bullet, also known as arsphenamine, led eventually to better arsenicals, such as arsenoxide. In 1921, bismuth, another heavy metal, was added to the antisyphilitic armamentarium.

Both of these, and especially the arsenicals, are now generally thought to have been effective against syphilis, but they also possessed serious drawbacks. As early as 1913 there had been at least 126 deaths from the use of Salvarsan, and it was estimated that there was about one fatality for every two thousand injections. In addition, it produced hepatitis, severe skin reactions, gangrene, and thrombosis and inflammation of the veins into which it was administered. The central nervous system and kidneys were also adversely affected. In 1933, a standard textbook stated that a patient receiving arsphenamine treatment ran a 0.3 percent risk of dying as a result of treatment (45). As many as 30 to 40 percent of patients suffered toxic effects of some sort. In addition, the treatment was a nuisance in other respects, requiring one-and-a-half to two years of injections, intramuscular bismuth alternating with intravenous arsphenamine. Not surprisingly, many patients never finished the course of treatment; at the famous Bellevue Hospital clinic in New York City, only 5 to 20 percent of patients were regular in attendance. To speed up the process, a ten-day blitz treatment was devised, but it required hospitalization and even then was likely to kill one in two thousand people from brain damage.

The confusions and misconceptions about heavy metal therapy came to a head in 1972, when the Tuskegee scandal broke across the news media of the country. The story had begun forty years earlier, when the U.S. Public Health Service set up an experiment involving some poor farmers in Macon County, Alabama, a predominantly black and illiterate county with one of the highest syphilis rates in the nation. The subjects numbered 412 persons diagnosed by blood test as having syphilis, 204 undiseased controls, and 275 others who had ostensibly been "cured" by the treatment then in use—bismuth, mercury, and arsenic. All were black men over twenty-five. Those with syphilis were left untreated, despite legislation on the Alabama books that said they should be treated. Apparently, in fact, when 252 of the men were called up at one time or another for Army duty, the local board was asked by those involved in the study to exclude the men from the list of draftees needing treatment. All subjects in the experiment received periodic checkups and treatment for nonsyphilitic conditions, as well as a yearly cash payment and burial expenses. (All subjects had agreed to an autopsy.) The trial was not kept secret, but instead was amply described in the medical literature from time to time as data accumulated.

Finally, four decades after the study began, it suddenly exploded, primarily through the efforts of Jean Heller, an AP reporter who got the lead from someone she met at the Democratic National Convention in Miami Beach. The fact that these men had never been systematically treated, even after penicillin had become available in the 1940's and was recognized as standard therapy, plus the occurrence of seven syphilis-related deaths in the experimental group, angered blacks and whites alike.

Dr. Merlin K. DuVal, assistant secretary for Health and Scientific Affairs of the Department of Health, Education and Welfare, quickly announced the formation of a citizens' panel to investigate the study. Five of its nine members were black, and the group represented labor, education, the law, theology, and medicine. HEW Secretary Elliot L. Richardson, addressing a meeting of the black National Medical Association, assured its members that the whole incident would be properly evaluated. The NMA continued its own probe, started before the government announced its policy. Retiring NMA president Dr. Emerson C. Walden called the Tuskegee study an "unforgivable, contemptible government plot of genocide" (46). The incoming president, Dr. Edmund C. Casey, said: "It's no greater a crime than has been done in practically every institution in the U.S. . . . First you try it in mice, then in rats, and then in blacks—because chimpanzees are too expensive" (46). Senator William Proxmire labeled the Tuskegee experiment "a moral and ethical nightmare."

Reporters alleged that the participants in the study were so ignorant "that they had to be rewarded and punished like children to get them and keep them in the program" (47). One of the rewards was being driven around in a large chauffered car with a government seal on it, presumably to allow the volunteers to impress their friends. The subjects joined Miss Rivers' Lodge, a combination social club and burial society, which met annually when a government doctor came to town. (The lodge was named for Eunice Rivers, a Public Health Service nurse responsible for keeping track of the men.)

Hostile comments abroad were added to the chorus of criticism. British, Italian, and Japanese scientists condemned what they considered an unethical study. Dr. Shivaji Lal, vice-chairman of the British Society for Social Responsibility in Science, saw the research as part of "a growing trend towards the use of medical power and knowledge against dissident and deviant minority groups" (48). He compared the Tuskegee subjects to Russian political prisoners and American criminals subjected to brain surgery.

The HEW citizens' panel quickly urged the immediate termination of the study, asserting that there was no convincing evidence that participants had ever been adequately informed about the nature of the research. The panel also recommended setting up a Select Specialists Group to supervise adequate therapy of the surviving subjects and epidemiological investigation of those who might have been infected through contact with the untreated cases. When Assistant HEW Secretary Dr. Charles C. Edwards released the panel report on June 12, 1973, he reported that all 112 known surviving participants in the Tuskegee study, scattered across fourteen states, had been contacted. Of these, eighty-one elected to receive federally financed health evaluation and care, five were undecided, and twenty-six declined.

Yet the comments were not all condemnatory. Dr. Thorstein Guthe, former Professor of Social Medicine at the University of Bergen and chief of the WHO Venereal Diseases Department in Geneva, recalling the classic Oslo studies in his own country, pointed out that the subjects were in general in a noncontagious stage of syphilis and that at the time of the study it was known that only one in ten such subjects would suffer lasting effects.

Dr. John R. Heller, a distinguished physician who once headed the National Cancer Institute and later the Memorial Sloan-Kettering Cancer Center in New York, was also moderate in his remarks. As a young PHS doctor, he had participated in the study, traveling to the sleepy little town of Tuskegee, examining the patients, and advising them on their medical problems. He could not recall whether the patients had been told they were not to be treated, but does recall telling his patients that they had "bad blood," a Southern rural euphemism for syphilis. Dr. Heller pointed out that at the start of the study, there was no effective treatment for syphilis and that mercury and arsenic were known to be toxic. He denied any racial implications of the study, but did say that after penicillin became available, he would have treated the patients (49).

The AMA president, Dr. Charles A. Hoffman, expressed similar views, condemning the failure to use penicillin. He reminded people that the treatment of syphilis was far from clear, even in the latter part of the 1940's. "Let's face it, penicillin had its dangers too. About 18 to 20 years ago we had something like 200 deaths from penicillin in a single year. I can recall that at one point we were told we should not use it unless absolutely indicated." Dr. Hoffman also referred to the questions of the availability and cost of penicillin. "I remember the first penicillin I ever saw was during the Second World War when the wife of a lieutenant was dying of septicemia. The air force flew in a vial of penicillin. . . . The cost of that vial was $5,000. It was not until 1948 or so that penicillin became inexpensive and plentiful enough to use."

Exactly what *did* happen to the Tuskegee subjects? How much harm did they suffer? The first published findings appeared in 1936 and reported abnormalities of the cardiovascular and central nervous systems and of the bones and joints. Ten years later Dr. Heller and Dr. P. T. Brunzere published a follow-up, reporting that the life expectancy of a patient who entered the study between the ages of twenty-five and fifty and received no treatment was reduced by about 20 percent. Eight years later the data showed a figure of 17 percent for those under fifty, 14 percent for those between fifty and sixty-five, and 6 percent for those over sixty-five.

By 1964, about 54 percent of the syphilitics and 45 percent of the control group had died. Twelve percent of the syphilitics who were examined had clinical evidence of late syphilis, primarily of the cardiovascular variety. The 1964 report estimated that 96 percent of the surviving syphilitics had in fact received some specific therapy for their disease, and perhaps a third of the group had actually received enough treatment to have been cured. By 1971, all but one of the subjects had received antisyphilitic therapy.

The most pertinent analysis, in some respects, however, has been made by Dr. Leonard J. Goldwater, an expert in public health. Long a student of mercury, he is more aware than most of the limitations in the use of heavy metals in the therapy of syphilis. Most critical analyses of the Tuskegee study have used nonsyphilitics as a control group for their calculations. Since syphilis can kill, it is not surprising that untreated syphilitics die on average at an earlier age than an uninfected population. But, as Professor Goldwater has so cogently suggested, *the untreated Tuskegee volunteers should properly be compared with a group of syphilitics who were treated by the then conventional therapy.* And what does such a comparison show? Life insurance figures for the period 1909–27 are available to shed light on this question. Syphilitics untreated or inadequately treated had a 141 to 142 percent mortality ratio (actual to expected deaths). *But syphilitics "cured through treatment" had a mortality ratio of 150 to 163 percent, substantially higher than the untreated.*

These data are not, to be sure, beyond criticism. Insured patients are not necessarily the same as noninsured. But the figures suggest strongly that the untreated Tuskegee patients—at least until penicillin was shown to be effective—may have been the lucky ones. This does not excuse the study's ethical shortcomings in regard to candid explanation of what was planned, or the failure to get fully informed consent (a procedure neglected by most researchers at the time the study began), but it shows that the desire of its planners to study the relative advantages and disadvantages of heavy metal therapy for syphilis may have been both scientifically and ethically sound.

The Final Report of the Tuskegee Syphilis Study Ad Hoc Advisory Panel makes interesting reading. The panel could find no protocol to document the original intent of the study. A search of the literature and interviews with study participants gave no evidence that any written protocol ever existed. A number of purposes for the study had been postulated from time to time and included the following: study of the natural history of syphilis, study of the course of treated and untreated syphilis, study of the differences in course of the disease in black versus white subjects, study of the hypothesis that syphilis in its later stages was relatively benign and therapy relatively dangerous, and study of ways to improve syphilis control programs in rural impoverished communities.

In a letter written by Assistant Surgeon General T. Clark to M. M. Davis of the Rosenwald Fund in 1932, it appears that a short-term study (six months or longer) may originally have been intended, simply to study the incidence and clinical course of late latent syphilis in the Negro male. At some time, however, a decision must also have been made to continue with a long-term study.

The committee could find no evidence that fully informed consent was sought, with full disclosure of risk both to patients and to others with whom they came in contact. This criticism was especially cogent to the panel because of statements in the scientific literature —possibly erroneous, as discussed earlier—that the benefits of treatment (including elimination of infectiousness) were already known in 1932 to outweigh the hazards of the medication then available.

The most compelling indictment, however, is that leveled at the scientific validity of the study. If the panel is correct in its statements, the Tuskegee study was doomed to failure because of its poor planning and execution and because of several unforeseen events. Since the "untreated" group almost all received therapy at some time, they were less than adequate as a reflection of the "natural" history of syphilis. There is also evidence that control subjects who became syphilitic were transferred to the "untreated" group, so that the study was (at least in part) not purely one of late latent syphilis. Finally, the absence of protocol suggested to the panel that systematic observations to evaluate the course of the patients were not made, and therefore no interpretable data were obtained. It is interesting that the data were good enough for many people to damn the study, however; critics seemed quite satisfied with the proof of *harm* to the untreated patients.

The least defensible kind of study is one that is a sheer waste, one that cannot possibly yield useful and valid data. As the panel states, "It is possible that a scientific study in 1932 of untreated syphilis, properly conceived with a clear protocol and conducted with suitable subjects who fully understood the implications of their involvement, might have been justified in the pre-penicillin era. This is especially true when one considers the uncertain nature of the results of treatment of late latent syphilis and the highly toxic nature of therapeutic agents then available" (50). Amen.

Perhaps the most important result of the Tuskegee incident is the response of the panel to the charge from Dr. DuVal to determine "whether existing policies to protect the rights of patients participating in health research conducted or supported by the Department of Health, Education, and Welfare are adequate and effective and to recommend improvements in these policies, if needed."

The panel concluded that these policies were *not* adequate. They decided this not only on the basis of the Tuskegee experiment and of reports from the 1960's of unethical experiments—all of which could be criticized as no longer typical of modern research philosophy and procedure—but also on the basis of a more recent survey by Professor Bernard Barber and his sociologist colleagues at Columbia University (51). The Barber group had reported in 1973 that "while the large majority of our samples of biomedical researchers seems to hold and live up to high ethical standards, a significant minority may not."

The panel therefore made "far-reaching recommendations for change." The main proposals were as follows:

1. Congress should establish a permanent body with the authority to regulate *at least* all Federally supported research involving human subjects, whether it is conducted in intramural or extramural settings,

or sponsored by DHEW or other government agencies, such as the Department of Defense. Ideally, the authority of this body should extend to all research activities, even those not Federally supported. But such a proposal may raise major jurisdictional problems. This body could be called the National Human Investigation Board. The Board should be independent of DHEW, for we do not believe that the agency which both conducts a great deal of research itself and supports much of the research that is carried on elsewhere is [in] a position to carry out dispassionately the functions we have in mind. The members of the Board should be appointed from diverse professional and scientific disciplines, and should include representatives from the public at large.

2. The primary responsibility of the National Human Investigation Board should be to formulate research policies, in much greater detail and with much more clarity than is presently the case. The Board must promulgate detailed procedures to govern the implementation of its policies by institutional review committees. It must also promulgate procedures for the review of research decisions and their consequences. In particular, this Board should establish procedures for the publication of important institutional committee and Board decisions. Publication of such decisions would permit their intensive study both inside and outside the medical profession and would be a first step toward the case-by-case development of policies governing human experimentation. We regard such a development, analogous to the experience of the common law, as the best hope for ultimately providing workable standards for the regulation of the human experimentation process.

3. The National Human Investigation Board should develop appeals procedures for the adjudication of disagreements between investigators and the institutional review committees.

4. The National Human Investigation Board should also develop a "no fault" clinical research insurance plan to assure compensation for subjects harmed as a result of their participation in research. Institutions which sponsor Federally supported research activities should be required to participate in such a plan.

5. With the establishment of adequate policy formulation and review mechanisms, the structure and functions of the institutional review committees should be altered to enhance the effectiveness of prior review. In place of the amorphous institutional review committee as it now exists, we propose the creation of an Institutional Human Investigation Committee (IHIC) with two distinct subcommittees. The IHIC should be the direct link between the institution and the National Human Investigation Board, and should establish local regulations consistent with national policies. The IHIC should also assume an educational role in its institutions, informing participants in the research enterprise of their rights and obligations. The implementation of research policies should be left to the two subcommittees of the IHIC.

a. A Protocol Review Group (PRG) should be responsible for the prior review of research protocols. The PRG should be composed mainly of competent biomedical professionals.

b. A Subject Advisory Group (SAG) should be responsible for aiding subjects in their decisionmaking whenever they request its services. Subjects must be made aware of the existence of the SAG. The primary concern of the SAG should be with procedures for obtaining consent, and with the quality of consents obtained. The SAG should be composed of both professionals and laymen (50).

These recommendations were received warmly in some congressional quarters, and a national commission was created in 1974 by Public Law 93–348 to study the ethical, moral, and legal implications of biomedical research and scientific advances.

Researchers have been somewhat less sanguine, for a variety of reasons. They point out that informed consent and protocol review are almost standard in most institutions now and that the excesses of the past are not likely to be repeated (although an occasional questionable piece of research still goes on). Some have criticized the inexperience of the Tuskegee panel in biomedical research, that they "don't know the realities of clinical investigation." Still another criticism is based on the problems that may be generated by a geographically (and perhaps intellectually) distant National Human Investigation Board formulating detailed policies and procedures to cover an infinite variety of research projects. Experienced clinical investigators are fearful of the ever-increasing complexity of procedures for scrutinizing their research, and of the stultifying effect of excessive controls on research that badly needs doing. To all this, the amateur and professional ethicists whose hackles have been raised by the Tuskegee and other biomedical scandals respond with a shrug and the assertion that society will inevitably be better off, despite any problems that may arise. Nonetheless, decision-making on the Potomac has in recent years been so often lacking in both wisdom and morality that one must worry more than a little over the notion that a Washington-based superboard will be an improvement over local attempts to improve the ethical quality of human research and safeguard the rights and bodies of patient subjects.

This controversy over one attempt to assess VD treatment is a prototype of the conflicts that arise when treatments in general require evaluation. Social needs and the needs (and rights) of specific individuals are not identical. At times they may be in direct conflict. The history of therapeutics is replete with examples of putative remedies that on critical examination turned out to be ineffective, unexpectedly toxic, or both. The Tuskegee episode, by dredging up past data on heavy metals, has reminded us forcefully of the errors of the past, both ethical and scientific. It is to be hoped that we can do better in the future on both levels.

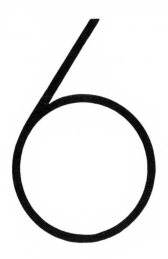

The Advent
of Effective
Therapy

In October 1943 the American Public Health Association held its annual meeting. One of the speakers, Dr. E. M. Mahoney, reported his results on four patients treated with injections of 25,000 units of penicillin every four hours for eight days. After sixteen hours spirochetes could no longer be seen in the lesions and the reagin which renders the Wassermann test positive rapidly disappeared from the blood. The audience broke into cheers at the conclusion of the brief presentation. What medicine had sought for centuries had finally arrived—an effective cure for syphilis.

The discovery of penicillin was the result of serendipity. Sir Alexander Fleming, his "prepared mind" ready to take advantage of the chance contamination of one of his culture plates by a penicillin-producing mold, had made his observations in 1929, but the practical application of the antibiotic had to wait until the early 1940's. The early history of penicillin was marked by two separate problems: how to improve on the original material and how to produce enough antibiotic to treat large numbers of people.

An early variant was benzyl penicillin, or penicillin

73

G, in many ways still a splendid performer. But G is susceptible to attack by the acid gastric juice and therefore treatment is much less efficient when this drug is given by mouth. Later relatives, such as the acid-stable penicillin V and ampicillin, did not have this drawback; their present status will be described shortly.

How does penicillin work? The antibiotic appears to bind irreversibly to microorganisms and to interfere with the synthesis of the glycopeptides that are crucial for maintaining the integrity of the cell wall, the bacterium's "overcoat." Stripped of their outer protection, the organisms die because water rushes in. This explains not only why penicillin kills microorganisms, but also why it doesn't harm animal tissue cells, which possess no glycopeptides in their cell walls. It is currently thought that penicillin exerts its lethal effects when the bacteria are growing or multiplying. For some bugs, there is reason to believe that damage to the cell wall may result in the transformation of sensitive microorganisms into resistant atypical forms. There is no evidence that such a phenomenon poses practical problems with *Treponema pallidum*, although a French worker named P. Collart has reported "dormant" treponemal forms in the tissues of patients with previously treated late syphilis. His work has been confirmed by several other laboratory groups and will be discussed later in this chapter.

T. pallidum is one of the most penicillin-sensitive microorganisms known. For penicillin to cure syphilis, however, the body fluids must attain a treponema-killing concentration of penicillin for a long enough period, and the body concentration of penicillin must not fall to ineffective levels for longer than twenty-four to thirty hours between doses lest the spirochetes multiply and outstrip the killing power of the antibiotic. From a practical point of view, these goals are most readily and efficiently achieved by giving penicillin in forms that provide more or less continuous levels of antibiotic for seven to ten days.

Penicillin G injections produce prompt and high peaks of antibiotic in the body, but the drug is so rapidly excreted that frequent injections are necessary. In 1945, the first attempt to produce a long-acting penicillin was made by putting penicillin G in arachis oil and beeswax. This preparation produced a lot of local irritation at the site of injection, however, and was replaced by a combination of penicillin and procaine, a local anesthetic, in oil with 2 percent aluminum monosterate, the so-called "PAM." PAM was better, but still not ideal, and was in turn largely replaced by benzathine penicillin, of which one 300,000 unit injection gives effective penicillin levels for about a week. (Eight times this dose can give adequate levels for three to four weeks.)

In 1949, Harry Eagle showed that the treponema-killing action of a given amount of penicillin was inversely related to the number of organisms present (52). Early in infection, with only a few treponemas, small doses suffice. Later, treatment must be more vigorous.

In most infectious diseases, immunity plays a natural role in combating the microbiological invaders. Syphilis is no exception. If penicillin is given in effective doses shortly after infection, the host's defense mechanisms are interfered with and the patient may be promptly infected again on reexposure. If treatment has been inadequate, relapse can occur, usually within the first three to nine months after treatment, rarely after one year, and hardly ever after two years. It is therefore important to follow a patient with early syphilis for two years after treatment. It is generally assumed that infection after adequate doses of penicillin represents reinfection rather than relapse, but the two are not easy to tell apart. The ease of acquiring a new infection is obviously directly related to the prevalence of the disease in the community and the sexual activity of the patient, and these are taken into account in trying to decide—sometimes arbitrarily—whether one is dealing with relapse or a new infection.

In patients with late syphilis, symptomatic or not, the immunological pattern is pretty well established and can only be modified to a minor degree by penicillin. At this stage, the goal of therapy is to arrest the infection, and blood test changes are of less importance, as will be discussed below.

Some experts believe that the symptoms of early syphilis have changed since the advent of penicillin. These doctors assert that one sees more atypical chancres, longer incubation times, and milder signs and symptoms than in the old days. Other experts disagree.

Recently the World Health Organization issued a report analyzing three decades of experience with penicillin in the treatment of syphilis. The three experts— O. Idsøe, T. Guthe, and R. R. Willcox—scrutinized the voluminous published literature and could come up with only 5,640 reported cases that satisfied their criteria for diagnosis and follow-up (53). What do these cases teach us?

If one treats primary syphilis adequately before the blood test is positive, clinical and serologic normality is seen in almost all cases when reinfection can be ruled out. If the primary syphilis is associated with a positive blood test, the test becomes negative in 93 to 100 percent of cases, depending on whose series you read.

In secondary syphilis, penicillin also produces excellent results. About 98 to 100 percent of patients end up with a negative blood test, and relapses are not seen, the majority of recurrences being attributed to reinfection.

The results are also good in early latent syphilis, but a normalization of the blood test is less predictable and may in any case take one to two years.

If one studies the history of these treated patients, it seems that late complications are almost totally eliminated by penicillin therapy. In the 5,640 cases analyzed, only one person developed symptomatic neurosyphilis five years after treatment, and in this case the treatment was considered to have been inadequate. The results seem unrelated to whether one uses penicillin G, PAM, or benzathine penicillin, provided one gets the drug into the patient in adequate amounts. Only a few diehards still treat with a combination of penicillin and either bismuth or arsenic injections. The therapeutic results seem no better, and the patient may die or suffer a severe reaction from the heavy metals.

All of this is most encouraging, but what about the efficacy of treatment in patients whose bodies have been exposed to the assault of the syphilis spirochete for years? This question is less easy to answer for a variety of reasons. In late latent syphilis there is nothing really to measure except the blood test, which is hard to revert to normal. In late symptomatic syphilis, damage caused by the chronic syphilitic inflammation may not be reversible, or the patient may show functional recovery as a result of nonsyphilitic medical care (digitalis for his heart failure, for example) or as a result of rehabilitative therapy. The older literature is also hard to interpret because prior to the development of the TPI test the diagnosis of latent syphilis could not be made with certainty.

The objectives of therapy of latent syphilis include the prevention of infectious relapses and late complications and the elimination of transmission of the disease from a pregnant syphilitic mother to her child in utero. The tendency to infectious relapses recedes dramatically with the passage of time during the first two years of infection and after four years this threat has for all intents been replaced by a tendency for late complications to occur.

The results of penicillin therapy of late latent syphilis are excellent in all respects except the reversion of positive blood tests to normal. The latter goal is achieved in 12 to 77 percent of cases, depending on the series (and almost certainly related to the duration of infection prior to the start of effective treatment).

What of the penicillin treatment of late syphilitics who are symptomatic? The first fact to be stressed here is that such reported cases are almost invariably the heritage of the years when cumbersome and relatively ineffective heavy metal therapy was all that was available. The most dramatic gift of penicillin to society in the area of venereal disease has been the marked worldwide decline in late syphilis that has taken place since the 1940's. In the past, a high incidence of early syphilis was invariably followed, eighteen to twenty years later, by an increase in late complications. This phenomenon was not seen after the epidemic of syphilis associated with World War II, and it is assumed that the prevention must be credited to the use of penicillin. The decline has been seen both in countries where penicillin therapy alone has predominated, such as Canada, Poland, the United Kingdom, the United States, and the Scandinavian countries, and in those where heavy metals have been used along with penicillin (such as France and the USSR). In many countries, the experience in the last decade has been that late syphilis is now seen almost invariably only after a patient has for some reason not been treated (or inadequately treated) with penicillin.

For patients with late benign syphilis of the skin, mucous membranes, and bones, the results with penicillin are excellent, although the healing of gummas is slow and may take several months.

The results in cardiovascular syphilis are harder to evaluate, since irreversible damage to the aorta or heart may have occurred prior to treatment. Even the hazards of penicillin are difficult to ascertain in such patients. They occasionally die suddenly after penicillin treatment, and these deaths may be attributed to the so-called Jarisch-Herxheimer reaction, a sudden explosive inflammatory or allergic response around the spirochetes in the tissues. Yet we also know that syphilitics with cardiovascular disease may die suddenly in the absence of treatment, and indeed at autopsy 25 to 50 percent of these patients have narrowing of the orifices of their coronary arteries, which originate from the aorta in a region often involved in the syphilitic process. With all these shortcomings, the data nevertheless are encouraging in the 1,168 cases available for analysis to the WHO team. In most instances the results over a period of up to ten years' follow-up were termed "satisfactory" or the treatment called "highly effective." Blood tests were mostly unaltered, however.

In neurosyphilis, the results are again encouraging. Progression of asymptomatic neurosyphilis to clinical neurosyphilis, for example, can be readily studied. A Johns Hopkins group observed 765 asymptomatic neurosyphilitics treated with penicillin and compared them with 457 patients treated with metal chemotherapy (54). Progression had essentially stopped three years after treatment with penicillin, but continued to occur in those treated with heavy metals. The worldwide experience in regard to clinical outcome and the findings of cerebrospinal fluid examination has in general been satisfactory.

A particularly striking difference between old and new treatments can be seen in the management of primary optic atrophy. Without treatment, this process invariably leads to blindness. Arsenic and bismuth not only do not halt this process, but also can have a marked toxic effect on the nerve. Penicillin seems to halt the disease process in 50 to 60 percent of patients treated at a time when they have only slightly reduced vision (nervous tissue that is already dead cannot be restored). The Jarisch-Herxheimer reaction can occur in the eye as well as elsewhere, so that rarely a sudden deterioration in eyesight can occur as a result of penicillin treatment. To avoid or minimize this hazard, many experts combine penicillin with cortisonelike drugs in treating such patients.

Treatment of late syphilitic complications, even when successful, is usually attended by a slow decline in the blood test titers. If the titer does not fall, or actually rises, retreatment is indicated. Only a quarter or so of late syphilitics, however, will show a complete return of their reagin-type blood tests to normal. The batting average is even less with tests like the TPI. It is understandable that doctors treating syphilitics would like to see all evidence of the disease disappear, so many attempts have been made to improve on this performance. Penicillin has been given for long periods, or in conjunction with artificially induced fever therapy, or after treatment with corticosteroids. Nothing seems to work any better than penicillin alone.

As a result, physicians have had to console themselves with the idea that persistently positive blood tests are simply the results either of persistent antibody production ("immunological memory") or of treponemes that remain in the tissues, providing an antigenic stimulus but having lost their virulence.

As we noted above, however, the findings of Collart's laboratory and of other workers have raised disquieting questions about the significance of spirochetes that persist in the tissues of syphilitics. Collart and his colleagues took lymph nodes from five patients with tabes dorsalis and transferred them to normal rabbits. In two of these rabbits, darkfield-positive testicular lesions resulted. (One of the two tabetic patients whose nodes harbored virulent spirochetes had received 50 million units of penicillin four months before; the other had been treated seven years before.)

Workers at the Venereal Disease Research Laboratory in Atlanta transferred material from the lymph nodes of forty-five patients with treated late or latent syphilis. In two cases, lesions developed in the rabbits and live spirochetes were demonstrated. Both patients had been treated as recently as three years before the experiment, although, to be sure, the possibility of reinfection could not be eliminated.

A Miami group has found spiral organisms in the eye, brain, and liver of several patients with evidence of central nervous system syphilis, some of whom had negative blood tests. Materials from some of these patients also produced syphilitic lesions in rabbits.

In 1970, some physicians from the Johns Hopkins Hospital reported finding virulent *T. pallidum* at autopsy in the eyes of a baby girl with congenital syphilis who died at twenty-two days of a separate bacterial infection (55). The mother had received adequate penicillin therapy by injection ten days before delivery, and the baby was treated with massive doses of penicillin for seventeen days after birth. The isolated strain was not resistant to penicillin, interestingly enough. Since the spirochetes were absent from other tissues, it is possible that those in the eye had not been killed because of the difficulty of getting penicillin into the eye chambers.

Other clinical reports in the last few years also constitute a minority report against the generally optimistic picture held almost universally about the efficacy of penicillin in all cases of syphilis. Dr. E. C. Wilner of the National Institute of Neurological Diseases and Stroke reports that nearly a third of patients with general paresis showed new signs of progressive disease after treatment had presumably arrested the disease process (56). Dr. Wilner says that these data either reflect neurosyphilitic progression or increased susceptibility to other neurological disease and that in either case the prognosis for such patients may be gloomier than is generally assumed to be the case.

A Virginia research team has also reported "relentless deterioration" in five of eighty-nine patients with general paresis followed for over two years after treatment (57). An Australian public health worker came up with further depressing news in 1972: in 460 cases of treated syphilis, 10 percent of primary cases and 16 percent of secondary cases failed to show negativity of reagin-type blood tests after adequate treatment (58). He concluded that the sensitivity of *T. pallidum* to penicillin might be decreasing, perhaps as a result of inadequate treatment with penicillin or other antibiotics.

It is difficult to know what to make of these reports. One of the groups has retracted some earlier findings because etch and water marks on glass slides were found occasionally to be misleading in immunofluorescent staining for spirochetes. Other workers say that they cannot distinguish between harmless treponemes and *T. pallidum.* Some British investigators have found treponema-like forms in the eye of a control patient who had multiple sclerosis but no evidence or history of syphilis. There does seem to be more or less general agreement in regard to one aspect of therapy: once adequate penicillin therapy has been given, vigorous attempts to reverse persistently positive blood tests make little sense, since they neither achieve the reversion nor change prognosis.

From early in the history of penicillin, it was evident

that the antibiotic could produce generally excellent results in maternal syphilis. Penicillin is not only at least as good as metal therapy, but is safer for the mother and the unborn child and can be given effectively in late pregnancy when there is not enough time for heavy metal therapy to work. If adequate penicillin therapy is given, a nonsyphilitic child is born in practically all instances.

To prevent congenital syphilis, therefore, requires routine blood testing of all pregnant women, followed by penicillin treatment of all infected women and follow-up observations of their babies. Some developing countries continue to report neonatal deaths from syphilis, but this seems to reflect poor blood-testing programs.

The rare failures of prenatal treatment with penicillin are thought usually to be due either to a maternal infection acquired toward the end of pregnancy or to insufficient periods of time for follow-up of infants with positive blood tests. If a child is born with a positive blood test, and his mother has suspicious-looking lesions, she should be considered to have had syphilis even though her blood test earlier in pregnancy was negative. In Chapter 4, we discussed the problem of passive transfer of antibodies from mother to child and how this can confuse diagnosis.

There is disagreement about what to do if a pregnant woman has had syphilis in the past and has already been treated adequately with penicillin. Some would leave her alone if her blood test is negative or of low titer. Others would treat the woman during every subsequent pregnancy *regardless* of previous treatment or status of the blood. Obviously if the woman shows clinical relapse or reinfection, there is no disagreement: she is then fully treated again.

In early congenital syphilis, penicillin results in almost 100 percent cure of symptoms, signs, and blood. If a syphilitic child is treated at birth, the reagin blood tests become negative within three to six months. If treatment is given after the second year, the children (like adults whose treatment is delayed) are much less likely to show reversion of their blood tests. The extreme rarity of clinical or serologic relapse in treated congenital syphilis supports the notion that such relapse in adequately treated adults is usually the result of new infection.

Some complications of congenital syphilis, however, do not respond well to penicillin. In deafness subsequent to syphilis of the auditory nerve, there is little that penicillin can do, in contrast to the deafness seen in adults with early syphilis, where penicillin may at times not only improve but completely restore hearing.

The eye lesions (interstitial keratitis) and arthritis (Clutton's joints) are not dramatically helped by penicillin, which may indicate a special kind of pathogenesis for these lesions. This hypothesis is supported by the beneficial effects of corticosteroids in these afflictions.

As we have already seen, the treponema-killing effect of penicillin is related to the number of spirochetes present. If true, this means that "prevention" of syphilis by antibiotics soon after exposure should be easily achieved with modest doses of penicillin. As early as 1949 it was shown in a series of 256 persons exposed to infectious syphilis that 900,000 units of penicillin in oil and beeswax protected almost 100 percent against infection, whereas two-thirds of a control group with similar exposure came down with the disease. Similar excellent results were reported in 1964 in 748 contacts given 2.4 million units of benzathine penicillin or procaine penicillin G. (An intramuscular tetracycline preparation, by contrast, worked poorly.) Fourteen of 161 patients given a placebo developed syphilis.

On the other hand, we also know that a patient treated with an injection of 100,000 units of PAM for acute gonorrhea will have his gonorrhea cured but may come down with a simultaneously acquired syphilitic infection. (Three times this dose is known to cure early syphilis.) If there is doubt about the "earliness" of the syphilis, the conservative approach would be to employ doses recognized as effective even for full-blown primary or secondary syphilis—that is, a total of 4.8 million units of PAM or 2.4 million units of benzathine penicillin G.

To be truly "preventive," a drug has to be given *before* exposure to a disease. (During World War II there was a "Pro-Kit" with a tube of ointment containing sulfathiazole, calomel (a mercury salt), vaseline jelly, mineral oil, and cetyl alcohol. It was supposed to prevent both gonorrhea and syphilis, but probably worked poorly against both.) A single dose of 600,000 units of PAM produces an effective level for five to six days; a single 2.4 million unit dose of benzathine penicillin for two to three weeks. Experience in brothels has shown that repeated doses of penicillin can be an effective epidemiologic weapon. Oral preparations would be most convenient, but this is the least predictable route, both because people forget to take the drug and because absorption is more capricious than after injections. Nevertheless, tetracycline tablets and other oral antibiotics are widely used in houses of prostitution and by solo whores.

There are drawbacks, to be sure, of such prophylaxis: expense, side effects of the antibiotics, and the development of penicillin-resistant microorganisms (the gonococcus, for example) in the treated person. An interesting idea has been studied in Japanese bar girls who use vaginal foam tablets that also include small doses of such antibiotics as penicillin G, tetracycline, or chloramphenicol. The data are too few and the studies too short term for definitive conclusions, but the results thus far are encouraging in that effective antibiotic concentrations can be achieved in the vagina without significant absorption of drug into the blood.

The use of treatment in epidemiologic control will be discussed in Chapter 7, but we should now take up the impact on *T. pallidum* of penicillin given to patients for nonvenereal diseases. Since many tons of penicillin are used each year, some people with unrecognized syphilis almost certainly have their disease cured, or are rendered noninfectious, as a result of such happenstance treatment. On the other hand, the present tendency to use other, newer antibiotics for all sorts of infections (including gonorrhea) means that this lucky dividend of antibiotic therapy will no longer be available, since some of these newer antibiotics are of little efficacy against syphilis.

The follow-up of treated patients is of crucial importance. Patients with primary or secondary syphilis should be examined (and their blood tested) monthly for six months after treatment, then every three months for one year, and if possible every six months for the year after that. The spinal fluid should probably be examined at some time between one and two years after treatment, although treatment of early syphilis is now so effective that some experts consider spinal puncture an unnecessary discomfort, risk, and expense.

For late latent syphilis, quantitative blood tests should be run every three months for the first year, every six months for the second year, and annually for at least three more years after that. The spinal fluid should be tested in such patients before concluding that the syphilis is only latent. Unlike the early cases, late syphilitics do not necessarily need retreatment just for persistently positive tests. Cardiovascular syphilis is followed in the same way as late latent syphilis.

In neurosyphilis, most experts now agree with the suggestion made by Dattner in 1951 that one could evaluate response to penicillin by studying the spinal fluid. This is done at three-monthly intervals for the first year and every six months in the second year. The cell count and total protein in this fluid should return to normal, although spinal fluid tests for reagin may be positive at low titers for years without indicating activity of the syphilis.

After treatment of early syphilis in pregnancy, quantitative blood tests should be carried out every month till delivery. Newborn babies of syphilitic mothers should also be followed with monthly tests for three months and a final test (if all is going well) at six months. If the tests are positive and do not decline as predicted for passive transfer, tests should be done at more frequent intervals.

The Jarisch-Herxheimer reaction to penicillin has already been mentioned. It is not always of the dramatic variety described above, and can occur to a minor degree in any patient treated with an effective drug (such as arsenic or penicillin). A common form is fever, usually coming on a few hours after the first injection and needing only a little aspirin. Sometimes patients complain of malaise and joint pains; sores and rashes may flare up briefly. In patients with optic atrophy, paresis, or nerve deafness, however, it may be wise to prevent or abort the reaction with a dose of corticosteroid prior to the injection. The Jarisch-Herxheimer reaction is, sad to say, not the only drawback of penicillin, although this antibiotic is in general a nontoxic drug. (Except for the guinea pig, which is for some mysterious reason susceptible to penicillin, most species can be killed only if you give so much penicillin that the animal dies from the dose of metallic ion combined with the penicillin.)

Occasionally there are untoward reactions locally at the site of injection, especially with the long-acting preparations, or from the absorption into the blood of large crystals of penicillin, but most of the side effects are allergic in nature. Some two million Americans are estimated to be sensitive to penicillin. Allergic reactions occur in up to 10 percent of patients treated with this antibiotic, although in several large series of venereal disease patients the ratios have been of the order of less than 1 percent (59). Many of these reactions are only of nuisance value, like minor skin rashes, but some of the reactions are severe, and occasionally they are fatal. The types of reactions include hives, swelling of the tongue, shock, joint pains, fever, kidney shutdown, low blood platelet count, hepatitis, nephritis, inflammation of the heart, convulsions, psychosis, and death. Fortunately, the fatal reactions occur in less than 0.002 percent of patients.

Prevention of these reactions can be accomplished in a variety of ways. Penicillin exposure of the population at large should be kept to a minimum to avoid sensitization. This means decreasing the use of penicillin in agriculture and for food preservation, and prescribing the antibiotic only for valid reasons and not for trivial indications (such as the common cold, which in its uncomplicated form is not helped by penicillin anyway). The drug should not be applied on skin or mucous membranes, since this seems to increase the risk of sensitization.

Once a patient has had a penicillin reaction, he should not in general be given the antibiotic again. If in doubt, the doctor can do a variety of skin tests to help decide whether sensitivity exists. Finally, emergency treatment for life-threatening "anaphylactic" reactions should always be available. Such frightening occurrences require prompt injection of adrenaline and anti-shock measures.

Although penicillin remains one of our most important weapons in the war against the malignant cork-screw, its drawbacks have forced a search for other treatments. Some of the relatives of penicillin are of no use in penicillin-sensitive cases because of their anti-genic similarity. But a number of other unrelated antibiotics have antisyphilitic activity. These include the tetracyclines, chloramphenicol, erythromycin, and the cephalosporins. *T. pallidum* disappears from primary lesions within 5 to 120 hours after use of any of these antibiotics, although their killing effect seems weaker than that of penicillin, which in animals still is outstanding. The cephalosporins, being most closely related chemically to penicillin, seem to kill treponemes of sur-face lesions almost as rapidly as does penicillin.

None of these drugs has been studied as extensively as has penicillin, but most experts seem to consider their results in early syphilis as satisfactory; some consider them the equal of penicillin. Very few patients have been treated for prenatal, congenital, or late syph-ilis with anything other than penicillin, so that state-ments about the efficacy of the penicillin-substitutes in these conditions is even more uncertain. Nor are these other antibiotics free of disadvantages. They are more expensive than penicillin and can produce disease of the teeth, bones, liver, kidneys, blood, and bone mar-row, and superinfection with other organisms.

Before the modern chemotherapeutic drugs came along, the treatment of gonorrhea was most inade-quate. An infected man was given urethral irrigations, told to abstain from sexual activity, and drink as much water as he could stand. Eventually his urinary dis-charge and discomfort might stop. After a few years, he might have trouble urinating because of a stricture in the urethra caused by chronic infection, in which case he would visit urology clinics for the rest of his life for urethral dilatation. Infection of the structures associated with the storage of sperm or its passage out of the urethra could lead to sterility. An infected woman often ended up with surgical removal of uterus, ovaries, and tubes.

Effective therapy of gonorrhea began in the 1930's, when German workers discovered the sulfa drugs. The earliest sulfonamides were effective but moderately toxic; later ones such as sulfadiazine were therapeutically active, cheap, and reasonably safe. Unfortunately, the gonococcus was clever enough to spawn resistant strains, and therapeutic failures soon became frequent enough to render the sulfa drugs a disappointment. Then came penicillin, which until a decade ago was virtually unchallenged as the treatment of choice.

Before considering the drugs presently available to treat gonorrhea, let us discuss the factors which must be considered in choosing an antibiotic. To begin with, naturally, the drug should work. It must not only be active against the gonococcus in the laboratory, but must be capable of reaching the gonococcus wherever it may be in the patient's body, and in sufficient concentration, and for long enough, to kill the bugs. We shall return later to the problem of resistant strains of gonococci, since this varies not only with time but with geography.

Second, the drug should be easy to take. One that will work with a single oral dose or injection and that requires no further diligence on the part of the patient is preferable to one that must be taken repeatedly. Experience has shown that many clinic patients cannot even be trusted to take a second dose on their own after leaving the clinic. It is thought that a drug should quickly produce high levels of drug in the body that are then rapidly dissipated, because a prolonged and gradual fall in level may facilitate the development of resistant strains.

The drug must have an acceptable risk-benefit ratio. Some antibiotics are effective against the gonococcus only in doses that have unacceptable hazards. Other drugs are safe enough in ordinary patients but dangerous in people with kidney disease or in pregnant women. (Kanamycin is an example of the former; tetracyclines of the latter, since these drugs affect the teeth and bones of the unborn fetus.) Allergic reactions should be rare.

Because so many people have both gonorrhea and syphilis at the same time, it is important to consider whether one antibiotic will kill both organisms at the same time. Clinicians are, paradoxically, ambivalent about such a double-barreled approach. Some prefer a drug that hits the gonococcus but leaves the treponema unscathed, arguing that one needs to know whether a patient has syphilis because of the follow-up procedures that must be invoked if syphilis is present. Others argue that one can get around this problem by doing a blood test before treatment and again four months later and that it is desirable to cure both diseases simultaneously. (As indicated above, reasonably small doses of penicillin can abort an incubating infection of syphilis.) Still others take no issue with the above arguments but fear that routine use of penicillin to treat gonorrhea will sensitize people to this antibiotic so that its utility will be seriously hampered for such of these patients who later develop syphilis or other serious illnesses best treated with penicillin.

Economic cost, finally, cannot be neglected, whether it is borne by the patient or by society via health clinics and other public facilities.

There is at present no ideal drug that will satisfy all of the above requirements, but there are several that come reasonably close. Penicillin at one time seemed almost perfect, but several developments have brought other antibiotics into serious consideration as alternatives. Earlier we have described the tendency of penicillin to produce allergic and anaphylactic reactions, occasionally of a fatal variety. But in the treatment of gonorrhea, penicillin has shown limitations that have not surfaced in the management of syphilis.

In 1954, the most resistant gonococci could be inhibited in laboratory culture media with 0.2 units of penicillin per milliliter. By 1969 this had increased to 3.5 units. In Southeast Asia, some of the strains require 5.6 units per milliliter. In a Toronto testing program that involved 5,700 different strains of gonococcus, Amies found in 1959 that 63 percent of strains were sensitive to 0.01 unit of penicillin per milliliter and 98 percent were sensitive to 0.1 unit per milliliter or less. By 1966, 27 percent of the isolated strains were resistant to 0.3 units of penicillin per milliliter, and 8 percent were resistant to 1.0 unit per milliliter.

In East Africa, single-dose treatment of gonorrhea with 300,000 units of PAM in 1961 cured 96 percent of patients. Five years later, a dose four times this size failed to cure 18 percent of patients; by 1971, the failure rate was 32 percent. Thus far, North America has been relatively lucky, because practically all the "resistant" strains in our part of the world are inhibited by concentrations of penicillin that are readily achieved in practice. In the Scandinavian countries, there has actually been a *decrease* in resistance to penicillin, making one wonder whether the Swedes are perhaps avoiding trouble by treating patients more adequately to begin with. There is a possibility that the resistant strains seen in Southeast Asia may also be related to the availability of black-market penicillin and inadequate self-dosing.

What is the recommended penicillin treatment regimen today? For gonorrhea of the uncomplicated variety in both males and females, it is now advised that 4.8

million units of procaine penicillin G be given, half at each of two intramuscular sites, at the same treatment session. (These doses are higher than they were a few years ago; if the gonococcus keeps getting more resistant, it won't be possible to get enough into the buttocks at a single visit.) It is also believed that everyone should also receive one gram of probenecid by mouth at least thirty minutes before the injection. Probenecid is related to the sulfa drugs chemically, but has no antibacterial effect per se. It is used, rather, to compete with penicillin for excretion by the kidney tubules. The two drugs fight for the attention of the kidney cells, and probenecid wins, thus delaying the active excretion of penicillin from the body.

If one is to use an oral preparation, the Center for Disease Control in Atlanta recommends ampicillin, 3.5 grams, with 1 gram of probenecid given simultaneously. (In 1973 the FDA approved a special soluble powder containing the two drugs in these amounts. The patient pours water into a small bottle containing the powder, then drinks the solution.) For those allergic to penicillin, ampicillin, probenecid, or other sulfa drugs, one can give spectinomycin in one intramuscular injection, 2 grams for men and 4 for women, or tetracycline by mouth, 1.5 grams initially, followed by 0.5 grams four times a day for four days, to a total of 9 grams. (This assumes that the patient will take the drug reliably.) Spectinomycin is inactive against syphilis.

The cephalosporins are related to penicillin and therefore not useful in patients with allergies to the latter drug. They seem less effective anyway. Kanamycin is effective but damages the kidneys and can produce deafness. Erythromycin, which also has activity against syphilis, will cure gonorrhea if the drug is taken repeatedly over several days. Doxycycline, in two 0.3-gram doses taken by mouth one hour apart, has achieved excellent cure rates in early trials (60).

Thus, penicillin remains the favorite treatment for both syphilis and gonorrhea in many parts of the world, although benzathine penicillin and other long-acting forms of penicillin, which are so favored for syphilotherapy, are not advised for treatment of gonorrhea. In some countries, such as Sweden, Denmark, Australia, New Zealand, Canada, and Austria, the favored form of therapy for gonorrhea is now a combination of plain penicillin G plus procaine penicillin G, with or without probenecid.

All of the above applies only to *uncomplicated* gonorrhea. For those few patients (less than 1 percent) who have gonococcal arthritis, pelvic inflammatory disease, infection of the rectum, blood-stream invasion, heart-valve infection, or meningitis, it is recommended that treatment consist of 5 to 10 million units (or more) of penicillin daily for ten days or longer, and that they should be in a hospital during this time. Fortunately, such disseminated gonococcal disease seems empirically to be caused by bugs that are not resistant to antibiotics (61).

One final disturbing note about gonococcal eradication: spectinomycin, which seems great for eradicating genitourinary gonorrhea, has been disappointing in treating infection of the pharynx, and the same deficiency has been reported for the combination of ampicillin and probenecid (62).

The less common venereal diseases can be treated with one or another of the antibiotics already discussed. Sulfa drugs work against chancroid and lymphogranuloma venereum, although they should be combined with streptomycin in treating the former. Tetracyclines are effective against both these diseases and granuloma inguinale as well. Penicillin, so useful against the two major VD organisms, *T. pallidum* and the gonococcus, is useless against most other venereal diseases. Minocycline, a new antibiotic, is effective against gonorrhea, syphilis, chancroid, granuloma inguinale, and lymphogranuloma venereum.

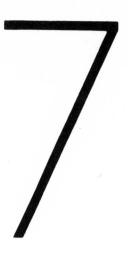

The Gift
That Keeps on
Giving

The fact that gonorrhea and syphilis are spread by sexual promiscuity puts them in a class totally unlike that of all other communicable diseases insofar as detection and control are concerned. People will talk freely about an epidemic of streptococcal sore throat, or meningococcal meningitis, or Asian flu. New cases are discussed with friends and neighbors, and health authorities are kept reasonably well apprised of the course of events. The public and the medical profession are inclined to work together to delimit and perhaps even halt most epidemics.

But VD? Hardly. VD is secret and shameful to most people. Nobody wants the neighbors or the girls at the office to know that she is infected, or how and when he got his "dose." The sexual contacts feel the same way. If the infected person is married and has become infected via some extramarital philandering, there are additional reasons for stealth, fear, or even panic.

To illustrate the epidemiology of VD, let us consider the account told by Dr. Nicholas J. Fiumara and his physician and nurse colleagues in 1957 in the *New England Journal of Medicine* (63). (Dr. Fiumara is Director of the Division of Communicable Diseases of the

Massachusetts Department of Public Health, and a frequent contributor to the medical literature on VD.) The epidemic in question took place in the Bay State, starting late in 1955 and ending (or at least slowing down) in the summer of 1956. The setting was a city with a population of 48,000, a manufacturing town whose citizens depended mostly on the employment furnished by the local shoe-and-leather industry and some electric machinery plants. The great majority (99.9 percent) of its inhabitants were white, and 85 percent were native born.

The first clue was provided by Alice, the attractive nineteen-year-old mother of a two-year-old boy. (All the names in this account are in code.) Alice had been unable to shake "a bad cold" and consulted her family doctor. She suffered from a sore throat, headache, low-grade fever, weakness, lassitude, swollen neck glands, and weight loss. She did not recall having had a rash at any time. Physical examination was not too helpful, and the doctor concluded that she had what was going around—a severe upper respiratory infection—prescribed aspirin, and told her to return in three or four days. Alice indeed had "what was going around," but it was syphilis, detected only because the physician was smart enough to do a routine blood test.

Alice had the bad luck to be married to Boris, a good-looking twenty-eight-year-old sexual athlete with dark, curly hair. Boris, the Bill Sykes of northeastern Massachusetts, was frequently drunk. During these alcoholic bouts he beat up Alice with much vigor and little mercy. Alice periodically separated from Boris but invariably took him back. Since he was Alice's only sexual contact, the search logically led to Boris.

Interview with the wayward husband required retrieving Boris from the local pokey, where he had spent the night after being arrested for beating his wife when she confessed a visit to the VD clinic. Boris resented

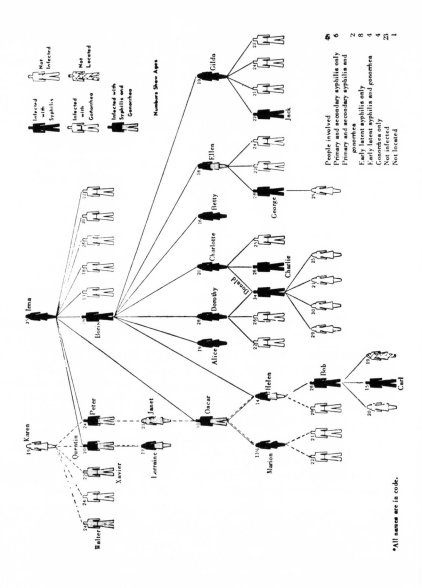

Outbreak of gonorrhea and early syphilis in a local community, Massachusetts, 1956 (reprinted, by permission, from *The New England Journal of Medicine* [256: 989, 1957])

any suggestion that his wife had dallied with other men, but volunteered several useful bits of information: a history of penile sores and seven sexual contacts of his own.

Betty, the first of these, was an attractive sixteen-year-old from a broken home who frequented bars and taverns and had had sexual relations with Boris on repeated occasions over a five-month period. Her blood test was positive. (She eventually became pregnant with Boris's baby.)

Charlotte was the second contact. A twenty-year-old married woman, she spent a weekend in town with her cousin, slept with Boris, and returned home with syphilis, which she promptly shared with her husband Charlie and a barkeep named Donald. She also made it in a car with a chubby out-of-stater named Edward, but Ed didn't catch anything besides Charlotte.

Donald the bartender slept not only with Charlotte, his wife Olga, Pamela, Ruby, and Sandra (none of whom contracted VD) but also with Dorothy, Boris's third contact.

Dorothy, a barmaid, was twenty-eight years old and a remarried divorcee who had introduced the visiting Charlotte to Boris. A swinger despite her schoolmarm-ish appearance—she liked to wear a white blouse with a collar, a black bow tie, and glasses with a black cord—she, too, was found to have syphilis. Her husband did not, nor did Frank, another bedmate.

Ellen, the fourth contact, was another child of a broken home. "Pretty but vacant-looking," she had an illegitimate eight-month-old daughter, gonorrhea, and syphilis. Two of her other sexual partners were free of VD, but not George, a tall, dark, and handsome, neat-dressing egotist, "with an aristocratic air" and secondary syphilis.

The fifth contact was Gilda, a nineteen-year-old who

left her husband, sought affection from Boris, and found syphilis, which she promptly shared with Jack, a twenty-nine-year-old bachelor. Three other sexual contacts of Gilda's were examined and found to be free of VD.

Boris's first contact, Betty, had an attractive fourteen-year-old sister, Helen, who was always in trouble with the police for truancy. She, too, had sexual intercourse with busy Boris, and was found to have both gonorrhea and syphilis. Helen gave the names of three other male contacts. Neal, who took Helen to the city dump for their carnal exercise, was free of disease. Oscar, whose wife was "frigid," had both venereal diseases; Janet, a "tramp" with whom he was in love, had gonorrhea. An eighth-grade student named Marion, who had slept with Oscar, was diagnosed as having early latent syphilis. Marion's two other contacts were free of VD. Oscar's last sexual partner was Irma, of whom more anon.

Helen also slept with Bob, a twenty-six-year-old who lived with his widowed mother and was very friendly with a fifteen-year-old boy named Carl. Carl turned out to have syphilis. Bob went to a private doctor with a rash and sores on his buttocks, anus, and genitals, and was found to have secondary syphilis.

Irma, the seventh of Boris's conquests, was an attractive, well-built thirty-nine-year-old widow with six legitimate and three illegitimate children. Irma lived in the slums and serviced many men in the area, who visited her day or night, were never turned away, and were never asked to pay. She was found to have syphilis. Besides Boris and Oscar, Irma named seven male contacts.

Quentin, her son-in-law, had both gonorrhea and syphilis, as did his wife. He also named Karen as a contact. Karen, a nineteen-year-old, had gonorrhea, as did three of the four other contacts she named.

Irma's friend Peter was a good-looking twenty-four-year-old who liked to drink and fight and who contracted both gonorrhea and syphilis. Robert was the father of one of Irma's three illegitimate children, but was free of VD. The four other males, ranging in age from eighteen to twenty-two, were not infected.

This spiderweb of co-op sex illustrates the way VD epidemiologic searches are conducted. Each patient diagnosed as suffering from VD is interviewed by skilled public-health personnel, who are trained to solicit highly personal information (in a manner that encourages trust in the use to which the information will be put) as to sexual contacts to whom they were exposed during the time of infectivity. For gonorrhea in men, the maximum incubation period is two weeks, but for women, because of the difficulty in knowing when this disease begins, data are obtained for all contacts within a month of the date of exposure. Contacts are also interviewed for the period after onset of symptoms until treatment can be expected to have rendered the lead case noninfectious. For syphilis, the incubation period is assumed to be three months at maximum for the primary stage and six months for the secondary. Those with early latent syphilis are arbitrarily questioned for contacts during the past year.

There is another approach, known as "cluster testing," which involves interviewing people named not as sexual contacts but as people who might benefit from an exam for VD. This has some advantages; it names people without specifying actual sexual contact and also involves people who may be at high risk even if they were not recently engaged in sexual intercourse with the lead case.

The account also illustrates the deficiency in this sort of case-finding: the failure to elicit a complete story of sexual contacts. Ellen, for instance, had both syphilis and gonorrhea, yet none of her contacts had gonorrhea. Who was the source of *her* infection? The information about Irma suggests that her nine contacts were far from the complete story. The account also shows how lost one would be in diagnosing syphilis without a blood test, since so many syphilitics are infected but lack either signs or symptoms.

The Massachusetts health team decided that the syphilis outbreak was most likely to have originated with Irma, the friendly widow, and that Karen was the fountainhead for the epidemic of gonorrhea. (Both women of course had acquired *their* initial infection from someone else, but the trail stopped with them.) The final score was fourteen patients with syphilis only, four with gonorrhea only, and six with both diseases. Twenty-three named contacts were not infected, and one contact could not be located. None of this would have been uncovered, and few of the infected patients would have been treated, if the first doctor had not done a routine blood test for syphilis and if the public health team had not been standing by, ready for expert interview, diagnosis, and treatment.

A final depressing note about this lower socioeconomic group of sexually promiscuous gin-mill devotees: by the time the report was written, several of them had already acquired reinfection with VD. In individuals who enjoy a varied sexual fare, with frequent intercourse with different partners, it is common for the spread of VD to keep ahead of diagnosis and treatment. Such mutual reinfection has led to the term "ping pong" syphilis or "ping pong" gonorrhea.

The rapid spread of VD is by no means limited to the lower classes. Dr. Fiumara has also described the story of "John" and "Joe," university instructors in the Boston area (64). When first seen, both had syphilis. They were roommates and lovers. John had acquired his infection "extramaritally" and then infected Joe. All three men were treated, came back for checkups, and referred many other worried friends for examination.

At the beginning of the next academic year, they came in again. This time John had a urethral infection and Joe had both a sore throat and a sore rectum. Gonococci were cultured from John's urethra and Joe's rectum and throat. Joe denied sexual relations with anyone besides John, but John admitted to intercourse with another instructor, Fred, who had come recently from the West Coast, where he had been treated for gonococcal infection of the rectum, which he thought had been cured because the rectal discomfort and the blood, pus, and mucus in his stools had disappeared. A specimen taken from the rectum was sent to the laboratory and grew out gonococci.

It is clear that exposure to someone infected with VD is not guaranteed to produce disease. Dr. J. Earle Moore, the late doyen of American venereology, once told me of a Marine sergeant who came to him with his first bout of VD after patronizing whorehouses for years in most parts of the world. "Doc," he said, "I've fucked them in Manila, Hong Kong, and Egypt. I've fucked them when they had chancres as thick as bees. And this is the first dose I've ever had."

How infectious *are* gonorrhea and syphilis? Reliable data on this point are not easy to come by, for obvious reasons. During World War II the U.S. Army did some studies with soldier volunteers in which uninfected men were systematically exposed to grossly infected prostitutes, and found that many of the soldiers did not come down with the disease. Fear of public outcry kept the lid on the results of this experiment.

In Singapore, in 1950, it was found that three-fourths of the prostitutes sampled had VD. Male patrons were surveyed as well, and 194 men were found infected. Of these men, 20 percent averaged one sexual exposure a month, 29 percent two a month, and 20 percent two a month. Some 154 other men were studied, of whom only 3 percent were infected during their first exposure. Fifteen percent became infected after less than ten sexual contacts, 40 percent got VD as late as the fortieth exposure, and up to one hundred exposures were without harm to a third of the men.

For syphilis alone, estimates range from 11 to 30 percent as to the risk of contracting the disease after intercourse with a floridly infected partner. For gonorrhea, the most recent data come from the study of an aircraft-carrier crew visiting Subic Bay in the Philippines for six days (65). The crew consorted with the 4,800 licensed hostesses in Olongapo, a town bordering on the naval base, and the rapidly increasing number of gonorrhea cases among the sailors prompted an investigation.

The hostesses were required to report weekly for bacteriologic survey, and one in five was found to be infected with gonorrhea. Eighty-eight cases of acute gonorrhea were seen—all in enlisted men. But 2,191 men admitted, by questionnaire, to contact during the six-day liberty period, with an average of three exposures. Only 23 percent of the men were estimated to have used condoms, and none admitted to self-treatment or antibiotic prophylaxis.

If infection were guaranteed by one sexual act with an infected partner, 399 cases of gonorrhea should have occurred, instead of the 88 actually seen. It was further estimated that the risk of infection for a man who had sexual intercourse 2.5 times with a given asymptomatic infected woman—this was the actual average number per consort, since some men patronized more than one prostitute—was 22 percent. Since not every hostess was infected, the risk from the same number of exposures to any Olongapo hostess selected at random over a six-day period was estimated at 4.3 percent.

While one can find experts who believe that the risk of contracting gonorrhea at a single intercourse with an infected person averages about 5 percent, this view is by no means universally held. Back in the 1940's, a Copenhagen study concluded that the figure was 85 percent or better, and at least one North American study put it at 75 percent for women and 88.5 percent for men (66).

Since epidemiologic tracing is not inexpensive, public health personnel have been understandably interested in the cost analysis of the various ways in which one might track down new cases. The Center for Disease Control reported, in 1972, the results of interviewing 7,353 men and 2,273 women with gonorrhea in certain areas of Alabama, Kentucky, Michigan, Ohio, Tennessee, and Virginia (67). The most effective way to discover untreated cases of gonorrhea turned out to be the interviewing of male volunteers who voluntarily sought examination. The cost per each new case in this group brought to treatment was $6.16. (Only 61 percent of these men had symptoms of gonorrhea.) The second most efficient way, costing $7.04 per each new case, was to study women who patronized family-planning clinics. Male contacts of gonorrheal women cost $7.96 per new case brought to treatment, and female contacts of infected men cost $13.60 per new case detected. Female volunteers cost an intermediate $8.04 per new case.

While one may argue about the value of new-case finding as a function of money spent, it seems surprising that not all states have gonorrhea epidemiology programs. In 1971, *Today's V.D. Control Problems,* an American Social Health Association publication, reported data from only 27.8 percent of the states and 53.7 percent of forty-five cities on interviewing male gonorrhea patients for their contacts, despite the knowledge that almost half of such contacts required treatment for previously unknown gonorrhea (68). The report contained no data on interviews of women for male contacts, presumably because most doctors believe that all infected men become symptomatic and will seek treatment on their own—a fallacy we shall discuss presently.

Many reasons are given for this lack of appreciation for gonorrheal epidemiology: There is only enough money to study syphilis properly. Without a blood test or a vaccine it's not possible to control the disease. Gonorrhea is too minor and too easy to treat. Gonorrhea epidemiology just doesn't work because the disease spreads too rapidly. And so on.

To refute these defeatist arguments, a team from the Norfolk Venereal Disease Clinic has presented some promising results (69). They utilized what they called "selective epidemiology"—a five- to eight-minute interview of male and female patients which encouraged them to bring or send in their contacts for examination or treatment. If this failed, the named contacts were approached by phone or letter, and occasionally by personal visit. The great majority of contacts named were actually located and studied (82 percent of 3,277 named). About half of the male and female contacts were found to be infected. Since this technique produced 41 percent of the total of gonorrhea cases treated in the Norfolk Clinic in 1970, the VD team quite properly concluded that it was effective and distinctly worthwhile.

Interviews alone are not adequate for either male or female cases of VD. We have already seen in Chapter 3 how VD, especially in women, can occur without symptoms or signs. There is increasing evidence that medical science has underestimated the frequency of such hidden VD, especially in men.

As early as the 1960's, symptomless gonorrhea in men was identified and reported by Dr. Harry Pariser of the Norfolk VD program just referred to. Its extent, however, is just beginning to be appreciated, as the result of large-scale screening of American servicemen returning from Southeast Asia. In one study of 314 men with gonorrhea, Dr. Frank Roberts of Memphis found that 20 percent had no symptoms (70). In another study of 2,241 Vietnam veterans, more than half of the forty-five infected men showed no sign of the disease. Frightening figures are conjured up by extrapolating these data: if this percentage of Vietnam returnees were infected and didn't know it, about seven thousand such cases were entering the United States yearly at the time of peak American involvement in the war (71).

As these studies are followed by similar ones on other male groups, it appears that Vietnam veterans are not unique and that men are quite like women in being able to harbor (and spread) gonorrhea without knowing it. The implications for the epidemiology of gonorrhea, and for follow-up of treatment, are clear.

Further bad news has come from attempts to grow the gonococcus more efficiently than in the past. These attempts have taken two tacks—looking for the bug in unusual places, and using better techniques for growing out the gonococcus.

The recognition that gonorrhea could exist in the pharynx and rectum, especially in homosexuals, has taught us that some carriers of the disease may harbor the bug only in these places and not in the more traditional genitourinary sites. The data also point up the importance of inquiring about, or at least considering, rectal intercourse more frequently than has been the case in the past. It is now evident that positive rectal cultures for gonococci do not generally occur except in those playing the receptor role in rectal intercourse. (For years rectal gonorrhea in women was considered a medical oddity, and complicated Victorian explanations were unwittingly fabricated to explain its occurrence: contaminated thermometers or enema nozzles, or migration of gonococci to the everted rectal mucosa during defecation.) To complicate life still further, much of gonorrheal pharyngitis and proctitis seems to be asymptomatic. Also, clichés about infected homosexuals being largely "arty" types have had to be revised as gonorrheal infection of rectum or pharynx have been reported in homosexual accountants, bartenders, cooks, doctors, dentists, engineers, fishermen, lawyers, printers, radio announcers, salesmen, social workers, songwriters, stockbrokers, and teachers.

Routine cervical and rectal cultures of women seen by one group of private obstetricians and gynecologists detected a 2.6 percent rate of gonorrhea when employing the sensitive Thayer-Martin media. A screening program by the Chicago Board of Health over a two-and-a-half-year period showed 7.5 percent of women from lower socioeconomic strata to be positive for the gonococcus if only one cervical culture was performed (72). In a VD clinic where rectal tests were performed as well, 24.4 percent were positive.

In a study of 702 Philippine nightclub hostesses, 8.5 percent were found infected at the first examination, but on repeated weekly cultures the prevalence of infection rose to 19.7 percent (73). Similarly, among 163 named female contacts of American servicemen, 22 percent were found infected at first examination, but the figure rose to 44.6 percent with repeated exams. Although the possibility exists that some of this increase over time might be explained by new infections, it seems more likely that the low yield with one exam reflects the considerable deficiency in a one-shot screening approach. The authors concluded that part of the variability was explained by menstrual changes; the best time to detect asymptomatic infection by endocervical culture is during menstruation or right before the start of flow.

Some British workers have compared the yield from vaginal cultures alone with that achieved by a combination of vaginal, urethral, and endocervical specimens. They found that nearly one infected woman in three would be missed if vaginal material only were examined (74). Their results are similar to those reported by other investigators and were interpreted by them as suggesting that the gonococcus does not survive as well once it is in the vagina.

A 1973 report from the Albemarle-Nelson-Charlottesville Department of Health and the University of Virginia suggests a simple and convenient way of screening for gonorrhea (75). Comparing urethral specimens obtained from men by metal loop or swab with the culture of urine sediment, they found that only 5.9 percent of urine cultures were misleadingly "negative" in patients found to be positive by other methods. If other workers can corroborate these results, the simplicity of urine cultures may be judged an important enough advantage to warrant their routine use in at least some situations.

In epidemiologic circles, there is an important controversy regarding the possibility of treating all symptomless contacts of patients with venereal disease. Advocates of such treatment argue that effective one-dose treatment of both major venereal diseases is now available and that treatment of contacts, infected or not, helps break the chain of infection and eliminates the patients lost from programs before a definite diagnosis can be made and treatment given. The data on diagnosis referred to above also suggest that reliance on simpler bacteriologic diagnosis may miss some infected people in any case. Dr. William J. Brown, one of America's leading experts, has called epidemiologic treatment "the most powerful preventive weapon" available to doctors.

Opponents of indiscriminate treatment of all contacts argue that treatment without diagnosis is bad medicine, poses ethical as well as legal problems for the uninfected person given a potentially toxic drug for a disease he doesn't have, and leads to needless anxiety and guilt. Unneeded antibiotics can also be counted on to incite sensitization to the drugs in some recipients, leading to allergic reactions and limiting the use of the antibiotics in the future for the thus-sensitized patients.

A further consideration is the time of incubation. Syphilis has a long incubation period, which allows time for the tracing of contacts. Gonorrhea, by contrast, can become clinically manifest in a few days.

Since only 10 to 20 percent of the contacts of syphilitics will turn out to have syphilis, opposition to "epidemiologic treatment" of all such contacts can be expected to be even more vocal than to the preventive treatment of gonorrheal contacts. Port clinics have long tended to engage in epidemiologic treatment of contacts of known syphilitics, but even there the practice is more widespread in some parts of the world (Central and South America, for instance) than in others (Europe, for instance).

Such decisions point up the need for balancing social and individual benefits against social and individual risks. In theory, treating everyone in the world during a given week might eliminate both gonorrhea and syphilis, but it is unlikely that the governments of the world would ever agree to this, even if it were technically possible to carry out. (In Chapter 8 we will see that this approach can work in a closed population.)

A number of serious problems make the control of VD even more difficult. Surveys show that only 12 percent of patients treated by private physicians ever get reported. In the early decades of this century, when VD was for the most part treated in special clinics, such negligence might not have been catastrophic. But today, because VD is so easy to treat, over 80 percent of VD patients are handled exclusively by private doctors. Such physicians are not only less adept at diagnosing VD than experts in venereology, but have neither the time, the training, nor the facilities for pursuing the sexual contacts of their patients. It is imperative, therefore, that the private physician promptly report the cases he sees and treats and thus delegate the public health responsibility to agencies capable of shouldering such responsibility.

Exemplifying the difficulties facing the doctor who *wants* to be conscientious are the results of a 1962 nationwide study. At that time—and the figures seem to be about the same today—25 percent of all sexual contacts of VD infected patients lived outside the city or county where the patient lived, and 13 percent actually lived outside the state. The average distance between the patient's residence and that of these out-of-county contacts was three hundred miles. Thirteen percent lived within one hundred miles of each other, 6 percent from one hundred to five hundred miles apart, 3 percent from five hundred to a thousand miles, and 2 percent over a thousand miles away. One percent of these distant contacts lived in a different country from the source case. Clearly, speed of tracing and a functioning network of epidemiologic experts are the key to success in such a situation.

The private doctor's role is not made any easier by the cultural restrictions upon him. Not only is VD generally taboo, and publicized extramarital sex a source of

potential embarrassment and legal strife, but the growing homosexual component of VD poses even more
serious troubles. Despite some progress by the Gay Lib-
eration Front in removing the social stigma attached to
homosexuality, the possibility of a secret homosexual
suffering socially by losing his cover because of the follow up of VD contacts is a very real one. I remember
the anger and hostility shown by an academic psychiatrist a few years ago when he was named as a contact
by a homosexual friend who was being treated for VD
by a private doctor. Despite the fact that the approach
was made with diplomacy and finesse by the doctor
(who was a VD expert), the psychiatrist rudely rejected
any offer of medical help and refused to discuss the
matter further. Sad, destructive of effective contact
tracing, but understandable.

Some gay meeting places, such as public baths, now
provide confidential service on blood tests. They will
take blood and identify it only with a number, so that
a worried person can call on the phone a few days later
and ask for the results by number, thus preserving
secrecy but getting information that can lead to effective treatment if needed.

Aside from the ethical responsibilities of the physician to maintain the confidential aspects of his patient's
ailments, he also has legal responsibilities. Since the
time of Hippocrates, the doctor has seen one of his
highest duties as keeping secret information about his
patient obtained in the course of serving that patient in
the role of physician: "Whatever, in connection with
my professional practice, or not in connection with it,
I may see or hear in the lives of men which ought not
to be spoken abroad I will not divulge as reckoning that
all should be kept secret" (76). This vow is elaborated
upon—and somewhat amended—in the AMA's Princi-
ples of Medical Ethics: "A physician may not reveal the

confidence entrusted to him in the course of medical attendance, or the deficiencies he may observe in the character of patients, unless he is required to do so by law or unless it becomes necessary in order to protect the welfare of the individual or of the community" (76).

The exception about what the doctor is required to do by law acknowledges the fact that the courts may require a physician to disclose information about his patient under penalty of criminal prosecution or loss of his medical license. But in the absence of such demands, the doctor may have trouble in choosing between the welfare of his patient and that of society and may have serious worry about the personal consequences of a court or licensing agency deciding that any release of information was improper. These consequences may include loss of license, action for damages, a fine, or imprisonment.

In one case, Simonson vs. Swenson, a doctor diagnosed syphilis in his patient but told him that he could not be absolutely certain without doing a blood test (77). Believing the patient to be highly contagious, he told the patient to move out of the small hotel in which he lived. The patient did not, and the physician informed the hotel proprietor that the man had a contagious disease. The proprietor threw the patient out. When the blood test finally turned out to be negative, the doctor was sued. The court held that the disclosure was not wrongful because the physician had a duty to prevent the spread of disease even if it meant disclosing his diagnosis.

Notwithstanding this precedent, at least one textbook of legal medicine advises that whenever a doctor believes it necessary to reveal a professional secret to protect the welfare of a patient, someone else, or the community, he should assure himself that the person informed is entitled to the information (for example, a parent or guardian of the patient) and, if in doubt, should consult an attorney (76).

On the other hand, the doctor is required to know the state and local requirements concerning the reporting of diseases. In most states, communicable diseases must be reported, although it is usually up to the state health authorities to specify which diseases must be reported and which call for compulsory isolation or treatment. For such data to be useful, the filing must clearly be made promptly (within twenty-four hours, for example, in New York and Michigan) and contain the name and address of the patient, his disease, its time of onset, and the doctor's name. There are penalties for failure to comply—a fine, a jail sentence, or both.

Venereal diseases must be reported in every state, and for these the report must also include the sex of the patient, marital status, whether pregnancy exists, the result of the lab tests that have been done to establish the diagnosis, whether or not the doctor is treating the patient, the possible sexual contacts, and whether or not these contacts have been examined. There are usually state health department forms for this information. Once the report is filed, the doctor's responsibility is over, but state officials can force treatment on infected persons or force examination on persons suspected of infection. (The latter provision is aimed at prostitutes particularly and in some cases is specifically limited to prostitutes.)

Premarital physical exams and blood tests are required before issuance of a marriage license in about four-fifths of the states. This usually requires a doctor's certificate of freedom from VD, but in fact the laws are oriented toward picking up syphilis rather than gonorrhea, for reasons that are not clear. Most states also require blood tests for syphilis to be run by every doctor attending a pregnant woman. If a premarital or prenatal test or exam is positive for VD, the doctor must report that fact to the appropriate health authorities. The patient may then be treated by any doctor or clinic he or she chooses. In thirty-nine states the law requires laboratories to report any positive blood tests to the state as well as to the doctor who ordered the test.

The doctor must report VD even if the information might result in prosecution or other legal action, as, for example, in the case of a young girl infected during rape by her father. In some jurisdictions, medical reports of this type have been judged privileged communication not to be divulged to local law enforcement officers, although some contend that the law only bars private individuals from such records, not public authorities. Society would be well advised to guard against misuse of VD records by unscrupulous men with access to such documents. In the wake of Watergate, privacy seems more than ever something that we will have to fight for if it is not to be lost.

Since syphilis can be transmitted by blood transfusions if the donor is in an infectious stage, all states require that blood donors be tested for syphilis. If positive, their blood cannot be transfused into a patient.

In the United Kingdom, there have long been specific legal positions about medical secrecy in regard to VD. The Venereal Diseases Regulations of 1916 state that all information from persons treated for these diseases shall be confidential. This principle was reaffirmed in the National Health Service Regulations of 1948, but in 1968 was modified to permit information to be transmitted to another physician or to a person employed by a physician in connection with the treatment of VD. Unlike lawyers and clergymen, who are never asked to give evidence in court in confidential matters, doctors are often asked to do so. Thus far, no British judge has asked to have VD medical records revealed without the consent of the patient. It will be interesting to see what happens if and when one does.

The sexual life of the young poses a whole series of ethical and legal dilemmas for the conscientious physician. Under what circumstances and at what age should contraceptive advice be given to a minor? An abortion proposed? Who should be told if a youngster is found to have VD? The physician is torn between wanting on the one hand to involve the parents so as to support the minor through a difficult situation (and to avoid legal and other recrimination) and on the other hand to respect the confidence of his young patient and maintain the youngster's cooperation in taking treatment and giving the names of contacts.

The presence of legal obstacles in the past forbidding treatment of minors without parental consent imposed a rigidity that was certainly harmful. Limiting the options of doctor and patient is usually undesirable in medicine—as in all other aspects of life—and it is encouraging to note that most states have passed legislation permitting doctors to treat minors for VD on the basis of their own consent. Only Wyoming and Wisconsin do not have laws stating that minors may be examined and treated for VD without consent. Even in South Carolina, Vermont, and Idaho, where the law states that parental consent is needed, there are opinions from the attorneys general that favor treatment without parental notification. Such laws do not oblige the physician to inform parents that their child has gonorrhea or syphilis, nor do they proscribe his involving the family if it seems desirable or necessary. Since so much VD is now occurring in the young, a more enlightened approach to the infected teenager should help society in its war against these modern plagues.

Some years ago I noticed in the Eye Clinic of one of

the world's great hospitals a notice describing the rules of consent for surgical and nonsurgical treatment. It warned that minors could not be treated without parental consent. There was an exception, however. If the minor had a venereal disease, the rule did not apply. VD had conferred what smoking, drinking, cosmetics, "grown-up" clothes and manners could not: legal maturity.

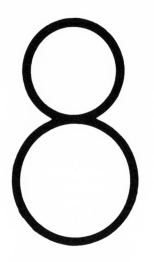

Past Hypocrisy, Present Ignorance, and a Doubtful Future

At the turn of the century, Mrs. William Bauern-schmidt, a civic leader of Baltimore who was executive secretary of the Public School Association of that city, met with Sir William Osler, one of the most distin-guished physicians of modern times. Sir William said to her: "I am going to tell you about a disease. I am going to give you the name of it, but you must promise me that you will never use that word in public." Mrs. Bauernschmidt, informed that the word was "syphilis," asked him to spell it and then to tell her what it did to people. His reply was as follows:

> It makes little babies blind, it makes people lose their minds, it cripples people. I hate to think of all the horrible things that disease does to the human family. I will tell you about it, but I want you to promise me faithfully that you will never use the word in front of anybody. You may mention it to a doctor, but tell the doctor immediately who told you about it. Never speak of it in public because people will think you are not a nice person, and men will tell their wives not to have anything to do with you. But learn from me what it is and go out into the world and try to help

118

and try with your influence and your money to do what you can for the human family. Never forget that you must not mention the word (78).

Mrs. Bauernschmidt soon began to see the ravages of the disease with her own eyes, both in the Babies' Milk Fund Clinics and at the orthopedic hospital where her husband worked. She decided that the parents of school children should learn about syphilis. The school board was fearful lest crowds of people descend on them "to protest against the use of indecent words in public" and destroy all of their programs (78).

Undaunted, Mrs. Bauernschmidt began, at first in one or two schools. The advent of the radio provided new opportunities, but the broadcasting studios refused to let her use the word "syphilis" over the radio. Newspapers would not publish the word. One day, to her amazement, she read in a magazine an excerpt from an article in the *Journal of the American Medical Association.* Here is how she recollects the moment:

> I read it and I could scarcely believe my eyes. I could scarcely believe it. I could see Dr. Osler, I could hear Dr. Osler, and I could hardly believe that the day had come when a man had dared publish that word and that the whole country, the whole world, would know that they could talk about that word and be decent. I thought about it and I felt a great relief and felt that, well, freedom was here at last (78).

These were neither the first nor the last evidences of hypocrisy and censorship in regard to venereal disease. When Henrik Ibsen wrote *Ghosts,* most of the ten thousand published copies were unsold, and the first production was put on not in Norway, not in any other Scandinavian country, not even in Europe—but in Chicago. Later staged in London, the play was labeled "putrid" and "an open sewer." The play, which deals with the Alvings and their troubles, ends with Oswald, the syphilitic son, mumbling senselessly, ". . . the sun . . . the sun . . .," his mind destroyed by the VD passed on to him by his father. The play's medical aspects are not quite accurate, but *Ghosts* remains even today a compelling drama with the capacity to grip and move people. For Victorian audiences, however, it was too strong a dose of reality, disease, and morals.

In 1901 another play about VD, *Damaged Goods,* opened in Paris. Its author was Eugène Brieux. Immediately censored, it moved on to Belgium and was allowed back in Paris in 1905. The work was dedicated to Professor Alfred Fournier, a great syphilologist after whom his institute in Paris was named. The dedication includes this paragraph: "I think, with you, that syphilis will become much less serious when we are able to speak openly of it without shame or fear of punishment, and when those affected by it, aware of the suffering they may cause in others, will better appreciate their duty to others as well as to themselves" (3). In New York the play was first produced for a private showing because of the timidity of both stage managers and actors. People who wished to see the play engaged in the charade of buying "membership" in a fund society simply by purchasing tickets. It was a great critical and popular success, toured the country, and was revived in the 1930's and 1940's.

Medically authentic—four French VD experts advised the author—the play concerns a young man with syphilis who marries against his doctor's advice, infecting his wife and baby. The marriage is wrecked. The key figure of the doctor speaks eloquently of the prudery that prevented discussion of syphilis and treated its victims as animals. He describes "the conspiracy of silence" that consigned the act of love to the category of unspeakable immorality.

Even in 1939, Surgeon General Thomas Parran was not allowed to speak of syphilis on the radio. On one occasion, a dinner guest of Parran's rebuked him for assaulting the sensibilities of decent folk with details of a disease that had been imported into the United States —along with communism—by "filthy Europeans," who deserved only to be shipped back home where they belonged. Parran reports that the gentleman's great-great-grandfather, an able-bodied seaman who had served on the *Constitution* and died of wounds suffered in battle with the *Guerrière,* is recorded on the surgical lists of the *Constitution* as having required treatment for a syphilitic ulcer.

As late as World War II, soldiers with VD were often treated for their disease in a punitive way, with a maximum of unpleasantness so as to discourage repetition. This attitude was by no means unique to the military; many people then (as today) looked on VD as an appropriate punishment for loose living by people who "deserve what they get."

If we are to diminish the harm to our society, therefore, such attitudes will have to be remedied. We will return to this important area of concern later, but let us now consider other ways of attacking the problem.

Americans traditionally are supposed to cherish the illusion of American supremacy in everything, although the success of Japanese radio and TV sets and of European cars testifies to our ability to recognize quality of performance in other lands. Are there any lessons to be learned from VD experiences abroad?

The first lesson is a negative one. High quality and availability of medical attention will not solve the problem of VD. Sweden, for example, has an excellent scheme of medical care which is freely available to all, but has plenty of VD. Nor does being inland, away from ports, ships, and sailors help; Czechoslovakians are abundantly afflicted with gonorrhea and syphilis.

Some of the Communist countries have high rates of VD (Poland, for instance), but Cuba and the USSR claim at least partial success in combating venereal disease. The Cuban rate for syphilis is nothing to brag about, but the country reports an almost unbelievably low incidence of gonorrhea. Since no WHO team seems to have investigated these figures or their meaning, it is hard to know what to make of them; no secret weapon against gonorrhea is known to exist in the land of Fidel Castro. The Russians report the opposite—low syphilis rates and high gonorrhea rates. On fairly careful scrutiny their approach to VD has not yielded any exciting leads.

The one country that seems to have achieved astounding success against both major venereal diseases is China. For some years now, foreign visitors to this ancient land have brought back stories that at first seemed too good to be true. In the mid-1950's, the collective reports from eight major Chinese cities listed only twenty-eight cases of infectious syphilis. In 1964 the occurrence of cases of early syphilis was reported to be 20 per 100,000,000 per year. VD was said to be so rare that lesions could not be found to show medical students. The reports now are too numerous and too much in accord to be dismissed as the puffery engaged in by an authoritarian state intent on putting forward the best possible image for international consumption. Where, then, are the answers?

We know that prostitution was at one time largely eliminated by the Chinese Communists, although the world's oldest profession seems to be staging at least a partial comeback there. We also know that the nation encourages what might be called an old-fashioned or "chaste" philosophy toward sex. Premarital and extramarital sex are frowned upon. Late marriage is encouraged, although early marriages are by no means prohibited. Divorce, however, is not approved of. Women seem to enjoy greater freedom of opportunity than in many Western countries, and the communal care of children provides more flexibility for achieving satisfaction in careers outside the home. Probably of great importance is the devotion of the Chinese people to the national welfare. The self seems largely submerged in the society as a whole. As a result, self-gratification and privacy both take a back seat to the greater good. Flouting of national ideals and goals would be difficult both to conceal from, and to justify to, friends, neighbors, and authorities. Such attitudes seem well suited to finding, reporting, and treating whatever VD exists. These attitudes may also explain another incredible achievement: the elimination of drug addiction.

But let us leave the Chinese and return to the problem of VD on an international basis. What means can we devise to decrease VD? Are there any simple, already available techniques that could have a major impact? Probably not, but we need not dismiss lesser degrees of gain.

Take the condom, for instance. It is fashionable to sneer at this as a protection, but such cynicism is undeserved. For the man seeking to prevent infection, a condom actually works unusually well, provided that there is no foreplay, that the condom is and remains intact, and that it is put on and removed with care. It is also recommended that the man urinate after intercourse and wash his genitalia with soap and water. The condom has limitations, to be sure, since it will not protect the base of the penis, the thighs, or the area above the penis, all of which may be moistened by his partner's secretions during intercourse, but "don't forget to wear your rubbers" may still be good maternal advice.

Because, in some states, young people have difficulty in purchasing condoms, and some people will be dissuaded from their use because they are unwilling to buy them, it may be necessary to give them away. The Human Resources Administration in New York City has distributed, through poolrooms, barber shops, and record stores, over five thousand condoms a month, free of charge. Condoms are also becoming stylish. The enterprising condom industry has come up with pink, green, and black prophylactics, and condoms in dayglow colors. There's even a variety called Tahiti.

Many instinctively believe that VD would be largely contained if whorehouses were put out of business or monitored regularly, or if prostitutes were treated frequently with antibiotics. Such extravagant hopes are doomed to failure, not because they are irrational, but because most VD is not spread by professional whores. Even if red-light districts were legalized everywhere and kept under strict surveillance, and the seamy "massage parlors" were similarly controlled, the amateurs— male and female—would still be out plying their trade, and the promiscuous of all ages and both sexes would continue spreading disease.

Nevertheless, Nevada's legal houses of prostitution are experimenting with progonasyl (an acronym for "prophylaxis against gonorrhea and syphilis"). This is an organic iodide acid in an oil base which when placed in the vagina and exposed to the moisture there forms a gel to trap both bacteria and sperm. Users of progonasyl seem to have less gonorrhea than nonusers.

That treatment of an entire closed community *can* work is shown by a blitz program in a southern prison housing over a thousand prisoners. On examination of all the inmates, 82 cases of syphilis were discovered. These named 209 contacts. To be thorough, every prisoner and all new inmates were given full "treatment" with penicillin. Syphilis was eradicated from the prison.

But all the world is not a jail. What one can do about sexual promiscuity, and factors that contribute to it, such as alcohol, marihuana, and other deinhibiting euphoriants, is not clear. Our nation, like many others, glorifies sex (not love, mind you) and ridicules chasteness and emotional reserve. Religious indoctrination is often useless because of a confusion of superficial trappings with fundamental morality. National leaders with charisma, trustworthiness, imagination, and courage are nowhere visible, leading to widespread cynicism and hopelessness among young and old. The family as a nuclear unit seems headed for the garbage can, with loss of parental guidance (which has too often been lacking or inept anyway). Marriage itself may be disappearing as a cultural necessity. Homosexuality, which is statistically more likely to spread VD than heterosexual promiscuity, is on the increase. (From 3 to 4 percent of American men are overt and continuing homosexuals, another 10 percent are at some point in their lives, and many more have homosexual experiences on rare occasions. Only about 1 percent of women admit to lesbianism.) Gay bars and Turkish baths make casual homosexual pickups easy. Travel is rapid and extensively engaged in, encouraging promiscuity that is not easily detectable by family and friends.

Can the Western world mimic China's cultural revolution? It seems unlikely, although it should be possible to make our society more satisfying so that alcohol, drugs, and promiscuity are not chosen in desperation simply because life provides no more attractive alternatives. Promiscuity is not a satisfying solution for the problem of an empty life. It is usually insensitive, impersonal, destructive, devoid of tenderness, and incapable of creating lasting relationships or emotional growth.

Respect for women, and equal opportunities for them, would raise the moral tone of our society. The same can be said for other disadvantaged groups, including the young, whose prolonged adolescence and failure to find useful cultural roles until too late, combined with a greater access to "facts" than their ancestors, have thrust them into a graceless pseudomaturity and maladjustment that dwarf the growing pains suffered by their parents. For too many, the Sexual Revolution has built a prison, not a paradise. No one wants to return to the psychological sickness that characterized past attitudes toward sex, but surely it is liberating to recognize that love is not the same as sex and to live one's life in awareness of that postulate. A lot of improvement should be achievable in our emotional life even if we cannot, or do not choose to, adopt a Chinese approach to existence.

In the control of infectious diseases, there are several basic approaches. While treatment helps those who already have the infection, and can decrease spread, eradication has usually been achieved by sanitation or immunization. But VD cannot be stopped by pasteurization, or killing mosquitoes, or chlorination of water. And as yet we have no vaccines against gonorrhea or syphilis.

Vaccines are most readily produced against viruses (polio or smallpox, for example) or bugs that produce toxins (like the diphtheria bacillus), just those infections that are not so well treated by the antibiotics available up to the present. But the major venereal diseases are not caused by viruses and do not produce toxins. Indeed, gonorrhea doesn't even seem to produce natural immunity in those infected with it. Syphilis, as we have seen earlier, does produce immunity, but the spirochetes are hard to grow and store, which is discouraging for potential vaccine producers. Despite the problems, work continues in the vaccine field, particularly in the search for one to prevent gonorrhea. Canadian workers have conducted trials in Inuvik, a community in the Northwest Territories, with a vaccine that seemed safe on the basis of both animal and human tests. Preliminary work on medical students had suggested that significant antibody titers would develop in over 90 percent of subjects. However, some subjects developed antibodies only very slowly and others lost them rapidly. The Inuvik trial was a total failure: ten of thirty-three vaccinated subjects contracted gonorrhea on subsequent exposure, compared with seven of twenty-nine placebo subjects (79). WHO experts predict that a vaccine against gonorrhea may be a decade off, although the recent success with meningococcal vaccine has raised hopes that the closely related gonococcus will also yield to this approach.

Inactivated spirochetes harvested from infected rabbits, in large doses given over a long time, have successfully immunized rabbits against infection with live *T. pallidum*. A cobalt source is used to emit gamma radiation for the purpose of inactivating the immunizing spirochetes, which are then given intravenously twice weekly for thirty-seven weeks, for a total of 3.7 billion organisms. The immunity this achieves appears long-lasting and complete. Attempts are underway to quick-freeze spirochetes and store them in liquid nitrogen, and also to see whether spirochetes given intramuscularly three times a week every third week will work as well. The research is encouraging, but there is obviously a long way to go. For the vaccine to be practical, science has to figure out a way to produce spirochetes in large numbers, come up with a practical dosing scheme, and then produce a vaccine that doesn't make human beings sick. If, for example, the vaccine contained bits of rabbit testicular debris, men might develop antibodies to such foreign protein and produce antibodies that could destroy their own testes. And if all of *those* problems are overcome, there still remains the serious question of whether the vaccine would render blood tests for syphilis useless in diagnosis and epidemiology. We rely so much at present on serologic help to detect syphilis and follow its treatment that a vaccine which destroyed the utility of all blood tests would be a dubious advance.

The lack of a blood test for gonorrhea has also stimulated research. A team of scientists at the New York State Department of Health laboratories has reported some exciting preliminary data. The test they have devised detects heat-stable antibodies to the gonococcus in a drop of blood by making them fluoresce under an ultraviolet microscope. The blood need not be freshly drawn, and the test can be done by a trained technician in less than two hours. This is in contrast to the present system of growing gonorrhea bugs from suspected infectees, which requires that a specimen arrive at the laboratory with the fragile bugs still alive and then requires growth of the organisms in a culture medium. The process takes anywhere from two to seven days, provided the steadily deteriorating quality of mail delivery by the United States Post Office doesn't kill the organisms before they reach the lab.

The first reports indicate that the test is close to perfect for women and about 80 percent accurate in men, who seek treatment earlier than women because of symptoms and may thus get treated before antibodies have a chance to develop. False positives have been almost totally lacking thus far in volunteers with no known history of gonorrhea. If present optimism is borne out by additional research, the advance could be a great one. The test's simplicity and ability to reflect infection in any part of the body would revolutionize mass screening and cut its cost enormously. Its major drawback is that it only shows that someone has had gonorrhea at some time, not that he has it at present.

These impressive achievements notwithstanding, the war against VD will not be successfully waged without first winning the minds of the people. Society has to acknowledge that the disease exists and that the problems raised by VD cannot be solved by secrecy and apathy. We have a long history of making disease even harder to control by encouraging people to deny its existence. Patients with tuberculosis or cancer have suffered needlessly, with delays in diagnosis and treatment, because of the shame that society attached to these diseases in the past.

Nor does it help for society to pin all its hopes on instant cures. Many of our medical problems are complex in both causation and remedy, and panaceas are not to be had for the asking. Drug addiction, like VD, reflects much of what is wrong with our society, and I have been distressed and angered on many occasions by parents at PTA meetings wanting a "1–2–3, you-list-'em-I'll-do-'em" catechism of how to "handle" a drug or VD problem if it arises in their family. We must begin with realizing that there *is* a problem, having compassion for those afflicted, and learning as much as we can about the situation.

Since one-third of VD in the United States afflicts teenagers, education should begin early. And education needs to include more than information about human anatomy and disease. It should discuss infinitely more complex (and interesting) matters, such as morality and love and responsibility. Youngsters have to learn that sex and VD are not only personal, but societal as well. Anyone with gonorrhea or syphilis should certainly have concern for himself, but he must also show concern for those with whom he has had sexual contact and who may also be infected. It is not enough to seek treatment for oneself; the contacts should be convinced to get treatment also.

The public should be fully aware not only of the magnitude of VD, but its consequences. Three-quarters of a million cases of gonorrhea and 25,000 cases of syphilis reported a year—and underreporting makes these figures only the tip of the iceberg, to be multiplied by a factor of at least 5 to 10 to get the true figure—is one hell of a lot of disease. It has been estimated that the United States acquires one new case of VD every fifteen seconds, and that one American teenager is infected every two minutes, and the facts should be well publicized.

The public must also learn of the serious nature of VD. Faith in antibiotics has somehow made many people think that a venereal infection is no more consequential than a cold or athlete's foot. As we have discussed earlier, prompt and effective treatment of VD can indeed cure it, but delays in diagnosis or treatment can lead to serious illness or even death. Gonorrhea, for example, can cause chronic prostatitis and urethral stricture in men and chronic disease of the ovaries and tubes in women. It is the commonest preventable cause of sterility in women and probably the leading cause of tubal pregnancy, because scars in the tubes prevent the fertilized egg from reaching the uterus. Furthermore, the antibiotics scene is not all that rosy. The gonococcus is showing increasing resistance to antibiotics, making treatment both more costly and less predictable. All antibiotics produce side effects in some people, some of them serious. An acquired sensitivity to an important antibiotic such as penicillin may deprive a patient of its use at some later time for a serious infection.

Another cost of VD that must be borne by society is the curtailment of life and the destruction of productivity in people irreparably damaged by these ailments. Each year two thousand Americans die of syphilis. It costs the American taxpayer over $50 million a year just to care for those with syphilitic psychosis in publicly supported mental hospitals and another $4.5 million to care for the syphilitic blind. Another serious national cost cannot be measured in dollars and cents but is nonetheless real and important—the guilt, shame, fear, and pain of those who get VD and of their friends and lovers whose lives are touched by gonorrhea and syphilis.

That young people are egregiously ignorant about VD was shown in the results of a questionnaire survey by John A. Yacenda, a public health educator and coordinator of the Ventura County Council of Free Clinics in California (80). Three hundred and two people attending a county fair in 1971 filled out questionnaires. Most of the respondents were ten to twenty-four years old. The responses showed large gaps in their knowledge. Twenty-five percent believed that syphilis could be caught from toilet seats, eating utensils, or towels. Nineteen percent stated that once the signs and symptoms of VD go away, a person cannot infect others. Almost three-quarters erroneously believed that you could diagnose gonorrhea with a blood test. One-fifth of those responding felt that information on VD was hard to obtain.

Those who stated that their information came exclusively from parents got more questions wrong than any other group. Those who received their information from TV, radio, books, newspapers, and the like scored better. No source or combination of sources, however, was deemed to be doing an adequate job. These figures contrast depressingly with the 1969 California law that prohibited VD or sex education in the public schools without the written consent of parents. In New York it is legal to include VD education in the public school curriculum, but it's not mandated.

The need for education is therefore unmistakable; the best techniques are not so evident. Programs are not synonymous with achievement. Exposure to information (or even the ability to parrot it back) is not the same as effective *use* of information. As Myron Arnold, a District of Columbia health adviser, has said, "Our purpose is to teach the student something he'll remember on a Saturday night, not necessarily on an examination" (81). Frightening people is not tantamount to persuasion; if it were, pickpockets would not have plied their trade in centuries past among those watching the public execution of thieves. We also know that a quarter to a third of new gonorrhea cases are "repeaters," and we have "educated" the public extensively about drug addiction without noticeable impact on the frequency of drug abuse.

Nonetheless, an informed public ought to be better off than an ignorant one. Wise decisions are not guaranteed by education, but they should occur more often in its presence than in its absence. So, the work continues —posters by health associations, pamphlets by college health services, ads by Metropolitan Life. *Young Winston* painted a terrifying portrait of the last days of Lord Randolph Churchill, as the once brilliant politician's mind degenerated in the wake of tertiary syphilitic involvement of his brain. (One could make a vivid documentary by combining film clips from *Young Winston* with the story of Al Capone, the famous Chicago gangster who was sent to jail for income tax evasion but who lost his most important fight to *T. pallidum.* He, too, suffered from tertiary syphilis of the central nervous system.) High school students, from all over New York City, have formed the Students Coalition for Relevant Sex Education to demand classes in sex and VD education.

One of the most imaginative approaches to education was the Corporation for Public Broadcasting's hour-long TV show "VD Blues," supported by a grant from the 3M Company. Hosted by Dick Cavett, the thinking man's master of ceremonies, the show combined entertainment with stern warnings. Dr. Hook and the Medicine Show set the tone with a theme song, written by Shel Silverstein, called "Don't Give a Dose to the One You Love Most." A Jules Feiffer skit involving a doctor and his infected patient was rough enough to bar AMA endorsement for the program. The best parts of the show were serious: a simulated documentary about a Newark ghetto and a bitter song called "Carrier." "VD Blues" showed that you could use documentary, drama, humor, and music to lure an audience, hold it, and educate without shaming. It was a far cry from the old Navy film that ended with someone putting on a rubber glove and admonishing, "If you're going to kid around, at least be safe." (Many a naive young sailor was confused as to how a rubber *glove* was supposed to protect you from VD.)

Although two Southern stations refused to carry the show, 185 of the 225 public television stations that ran it even scheduled special local follow-up programs or telephone "hot lines," which were perhaps the best demonstration of the impact of the program. New York's Channel 13 scheduled a VD hotline hosted by Geraldo Rivera and handled by sixty professional counselors. They received calls from fifteen thousand viewers. Cleveland's sequel ran from 9 to 11 P.M. and was rebroadcast by an ABC affiliate from 12:45 to 2:45 A.M., with doctors and counselors on duty to answer phones until 3:00 A.M. The next day, clinics reported a 50 percent increase in patients appearing for blood tests. In Chicago, one VD clinic had to close for two hours after the telecast because it was swamped with people seeking help. Philadelphia's teenage-run VD phone referral service, Operation Venus, received five thousand calls after the show.

Even with the rebroadcast of "VD Blues" six months later, its most ardent fans could not assert that one TV program, no matter how successful, is the answer to VD. Hot-line programs, however, do have a continuing role to play. The Philadelphia service mentioned above is only one of a number of programs started in recent years to answer questions and provide help. Operation Venus works exclusively by telephone. Never asking for the caller's name, the teenagers who man the phones give basic information on symptoms, causes, diagnostic tests, treatment, and where to go for assistance. They avoid making diagnoses over the phone, but urge all callers to get treatment.

In some communities, radio stations catering to rock music fans have taken to broadcasting public service announcements recommending treatment for all infected persons. Posters have been devised to appeal especially to itinerant hippies. Free clinics, some of them mobile, have been set up to cater to the special needs of youngsters disenchanted with the establishment in all its manifestations and hence more readily reached by medical facilities with less conventional ambience and staff.

At Syracuse University, there is a nonprofit center devoted to disseminating information about VD, sex, and drugs to youth in a way that makes sense to them. Realizing that a significant number of young people aren't interested in reading, the center has prepared a comic book about VD.

In August 1973 the *New York Times* carried a full-page ad sponsored jointly by the Alliance for Eradication of V.D. in cooperation with the New York City Department of Health. It urged readers to "fight V.D. with soap and water . . . WASH . . . an overlooked

technique of prevention. . . . Careful washing immediately after the act will reduce the possibility of catching
V.D. The proper use of a prophylactic is another way"
(82).

The educational effort cannot, however, be directed
simply at those likely to contract VD. We must also
educate the educators. If parents are to be effective at
the preschool level and later, they must be trained for
the role. A marriage license doesn't transform a man or
woman into an effective teacher, any more than the
scrap of paper prepares you to be a parent. Those who
are to teach about sex and VD in the schools, the
churches, the synagogues, the free clinics, the hot-line
services must be well informed. Nurses and public
health workers need to learn how to interview with
discretion, sensitivity and skill. The contact is rarely
going to be easy to deal with—he resents the diagnosis
of VD, is deservedly reticent toward a stranger prying
into his sex life, may fear marital discord, retaliation,
loss of status, or blackmail, and will be torn by his loyal-
ties to others. The epidemiological interviewer has to
overcome these obstacles and work with speed as well
as expertise, seeking people out at night and on weekends if necessary, while inspiring confidence that the
interviewer will not gossip or reveal the name of the
informant. The source may also have to be interviewed
more than once, since reinterview elicits new contacts
almost half the time.

The special importance of this part of VD control was
cogently put by Dr. Leona Baumgartner, former Com-
missioner of Health for New York City, in 1962:

The individuals who have syphilis have *got* to be
found. There are no if's, and's or but's to this. Finding
them will be a bother and a nuisance to some people,
but I think we had better agree on one point: if we

aren't willing to bother people in this matter, we aren't going to control syphilis, and we might just as well make up our minds to it (83).

Nor must we forget the doctors in the educational scheme. They are crucial in so many ways: they are considered experts by the public, they diagnose and treat most VD in their offices, and they are the weakest link in the epidemiologic chain. American medical schools, with their average of 6.7 hours for VD clinical instruction, 5 hours for theoretical instruction, and 2.6 hours for the public health aspects of VD, can hardly be said to prepare doctors adequately for the role they should play (84). VD, furthermore, requires a sophisticated holistic approach, since it encompasses sociologic, epidemiologic, and psychiatric factors, challenging the doctor at a level that is often not required by other diseases. If one adds to these troubles the fact that preventive medicine is not particularly appealing to most doctors and that many physicians fail to keep up with modern advances (a fatal flaw, for example, in dealing with a disease like gonorrhea, whose optimal treatment changes frequently), the outlook is not a happy one.

Dr. Philip G. Boysen, a Navy flight surgeon, expressed his views in the correspondence columns of the *JAMA:*

The concept that a graduate of a medical school is primed with all the knowledge he will need to practice medicine for 40 years is in a deserving state of disrepute. This particular dilemma further repudiates that concept. In my present status I have been presented with problems that did not exist at the time of my medical school instruction. For example, the relative resistance of the gonococcus to antibiotics has proved to be an increasing problem. The schedules for treatment of uncomplicated gonorrhea have been changed and the use of probenecid is now de rigeur. Spectinomycin was not yet on the scene and the need for alternative antibiotics in place of penicillin was just emerging (85).

Two physicians from the Children's Hospital Medical Center in Boston recently reported three infants with congenital syphilis whose symptoms were originally ascribed to osteomyelitis or physical abuse. The average doctor's ineptitude in this area can be measured by the fact that of 1,903 cases of congenital syphilis reported in 1970, only 300 were diagnosed in the infant's first year (86).

The United Kingdom is in some respects better off than the United States. The specialty of venereology is well established there, and most of the doctors practicing it are broadly trained in both the medical and the social aspects of VD. An Intercollegiate Committee on Venereology was formed in 1971 to study and improve the status of VD care. At least one university, Liverpool, has set up a special three-month diploma course in venereology. Since 1916 the national Venereal Diseases Regulations have directed local authorities to build, equip, and staff free and confidential clinics in all parts of the country.

Yet all is not well in Britain, either. Some of their VD posts are vacant and there is a dearth of young doctors going into the field. Venereology remains the only medical specialty without a university chair. Many of the clinics are small and badly situated, with inadequate staff of all kinds, from receptionists to social workers. Most of the clinics have no appointment system and are inadequate in waiting facilities and decor. When originally planned, these clinics had separate entrances and waiting rooms for men and women, to assuage anxieties and fears about privacy. Now, however, the "separate and equal" facilities simply discourage a boy from bringing his girlfriend with him.

Many of the troubles afflicting national and international VD control efforts would be considerably eased by an increased supply of funds. Money is badly needed for all sorts of things, including education, facilities, staff, case findings, and treatment. Grants should be freely available to medical schools to improve the teaching of VD and to bring the cloisters of academe in closer contact with the public health experts on the epidemiologic firing line. Schools of nursing and social work also need funds to pep up their activities in this field. Cooperation must be increased between federal government agencies and state health departments, and the networks of information at national and international levels upgraded.

And without money, of course, research will not be done—research on new and better techniques of diagnosis, contact tracing, and treatment, research on better methods of educating doctors and public alike, research on prevention of disease by any and all means, from discouraging promiscuity to prophylactic antibiotics. All of these are worthwhile, all cost money, all are at present inadequately funded. If VD is a serious problem, it calls for serious measures.

One of the most fundamental challenges facing society is how its quality of life can be improved. Urbanization has certainly been accompanied by increases in crime, addiction, and VD. The big cities of the United States seem to be dying, or becoming jungles. Deurbanization may not decrease all of our social ills, but the notion has appeal. Again, this will not be achieved without money (for such things as better mass transportation, for instance).

The Viet Nam War was associated with a great increase in VD among American troops. Its end will certainly not solve our VD problems, since the contribution of returning soldiers was minuscule compared to the contribution of the civilians who stayed at home. Yet the end of the war may be more important in another way, in diminishing the cynicism and unease among Americans who looked on the war as both foolish and immoral.

A societal concern for the quality of life of all our citizens may not eliminate VD and drug addiction and crime, but it is hard to believe that an improvement in the lot of our disadvantaged citizens, especially of the young on whom our future as a nation depends, would not ease our difficulties. And the nice thing about such improvement is that it's a "no lose" proposition—whatever happens to VD, the country would be better off.

Venereal disease continues to escalate. The incidence of gonorrhea in 1972 hit the highest peak in the fifty-three years since the U.S. Public Health Service started keeping statistics in 1919. More cases of infectious syphilis were reported than in any other year since 1950. Gonorrhea was up 34 percent in Omaha, 35 percent in New Orleans, 43 percent in Des Moines, and 44 percent in Tampa. Syphilis was up 31 percent in Washington, D.C., 32 percent in Boston, 41 percent in Detroit, 52 percent in Baltimore, 77 percent in Cincinnati, and 95 percent in Memphis (87). Both major venereal diseases showed still further increases in 1973. Nor is the rise limited to the United States; it is a worldwide phenomenon.

This gloomy state of affairs clearly calls for action. Are we providing it? What are realistic goals of achievement? What should be our national posture?

In a sense, we may be aiming too high. Our success in eliminating poliomyelitis has perhaps inflated our expectations to a point inconsistent with achievement. Most of our disease problems have not been eliminated by modern science. Many (like lung cancer and heart disease) are even getting worse. Some of the most significant advances have been in the nature of containment, rather than annihilation.

In many ways, VD resembles drug addiction. Both have been with us since time immemorial, and both are enormously complex entities that transcend the conventional disease model. The spirochete and the gonococcus are real enough, as are heroin and "speed," but so are poverty, cynicism, boredom, frustration, and the lack of national purpose.

Since VD is multigenetic in causation, it should yield best to multiple attack. A better antibiotic or a blood test for gonorrhea will not eliminate VD. Vaccines seem far off at the moment. But there is no reason to sneer at *any* step that may prevent disease, check spread, or facilitate treatment. The more liberal use of condoms will not solve the problems of VD any more than a new antibiotic will, but it could make a significant contribution to preventing some cases of infection. It is patently ridiculous to ban the Pill because it is an incentive to promiscuity, but it is not senseless to educate the young about the penalties for promiscuity and the difference between sex and love. Increasing the importance of humanity in our culture and deemphasizing materialistic gain, restoring dignity to the poor, reawakening idealism in our political leaders—such achievements could elevate the national tone in a way that might yield unforeseen benefits on the VD front. It may be no coincidence that the one nation that seems to have solved the problems of alcoholism, heroin addiction, and venereal disease—China—is also the one civilized country where locks are not needed on doors or bicycles.

The criticism may be raised that we *are* using many weapons in the battle against VD and are still losing the war. But it cannot be said that any approach mentioned in this book has been applied optimally in the United States, let alone all of them. I believe the war can ultimately be won only by the kind of all-out effort and dedication that allowed Lord Randolph Churchill's son and his people to overcome the threat of Nazi ambition. A reading of Winston Chruchill's six volumes on World War II shows that seemingly insuperable odds *can* be overcome, and victory snatched from the jaws of defeat, if faith in the ultimate outcome is accompanied by total commitment. World War II was won slowly and painfully, by taking many small steps slowly over a prolonged period. For a long time, no progress could be seen, but ultimately success was had by dint of pursuing the enemy in many places, with many weapons, wielded by many men and women, on the fighting fronts and at home.

The Battle of Britain and the war against VD may seem unlikely relatives, and analogies are always dangerous. But there *are* similarities, and it behooves us to ask whether we are taking as seriously as we should an enemy as formidable and relentless as VD. If we are failing at present—and it is hard to say that we are not —it may only mean that we are not as yet prepared to wage total war.

References

1. W. J. Brown, "Role of Public Health and Private Medicine in the Eradication of Syphilis," *Med. Clin. N. Amer.*, vol. 48, no. 3 (May 1964).
2. W. L. Fleming, "Syphilis through the Ages," *Med. Clin. N. Amer.*, vol. 48, no. 3 (May 1964).
3. T. Rosebury, *Microbes and Morals: The Strange Story of Venereal Disease* (New York: Viking, 1971).
4. "Venereal Diseases" (editorial), *Lancet*, vol. 1 (April 3, 1971).
5. "Undetected Syphilis Is Said to Affect 500,000 in the U.S.," *New York Times*, April 15, 1971.
6. "Roundtable: Venereal Disease," *Medical Aspects of Human Sexuality*, April 1971.
7. "Single-Dose Treatment of Gonorrhea" (editorial), *Lancet*, vol. 1 (April 22, 1972).
8. "Gonorrhoea" (editorial), *Lancet*, vol. 1 (May 20, 1972).
9. E. H. Hermans, "Interrelationship of Syphilis Incidence and Maritime Activity," *Proc. World Forum on Syphilis and Other Treponematoses* (Public Health Service Publication no. 997; Washington, D.C.: Government Printing Office, 1964).
10. F. L. Roberts, "Treatment of Gonorrhea," *JAMA*, vol. 218 (Oct. 18, 1971).
11. D. J. M. Wright, "Syphilis and Neanderthal Man," *Nature*, vol. 229 (Feb. 5, 1971).
12. F. H. Garrison, *History of Medicine* (Philadelphia: Saunders, 1929).
13. F. Buret, *Syphilis in Ancient and Prehistoric Times*, vol. 1,

trans. A. H. Ohmann-Dumesnil (Philadelphia: Davis, 1891).

14. A. Fournier, *Syphilis and Marriage*, trans. P. A. Morrow (New York: Appleton, 1881).

15. E. W. Thomas, *Syphilis: Its Course and Management* (New York: Macmillan, 1949).

16. E. G. Clark and N. Danbolt, "The Oslo Study of the Natural Course of Untreated Syphilis," *Med. Clin. N. Amer.*, vol. 48, no. 3 (May 1964).

17. E. Bruusgaard, "Über das Schicksal der nicht spezifisch behandelten Luetiker," *Arch. f. Dermat. u. Syph.*, vol. 157 (1929).

18. T. Gjestland, "The Oslo Study of Untreated Syphilis: An Epidemiologic Investigation of the Natural Course of Untreated Syphilis Based on a Restudy of the Boeck-Bruusgaard Material," *Acta Dermato-Venereologica*, supp. (1955).

19. S. Olansky, "Late Benign Syphilis (Gumma)," *Med. Clin. N. Amer.*, vol. 48, no. 3 (May 1964).

20. "Toilet Seat Gonorrhea Spread Reported by Swedish Doctor," *Medical Tribune*, March 14, 1973.

21. T. Elmros and P-Å. Larsson, "Survival of Gonococci outside the Body," *Brit. Med. J.*, vol. 1 (May 13, 1972).

22. Z. A. Sayeed, U. Bhaduri, E. Howell, and H. L. Meyers Jr., "Gonococcal Meningitis: A Review," *JAMA*, vol. 219 (March 27, 1972).

23. C. B. S. Schofield and R. A. Shanks, "Gonococcal Ophthalmia Neonatorum despite Treatment with Antibacterial Eye-Drops," *Brit. Med. J.*, vol. 1 (Jan. 30, 1971).

24. T. R. Thompson, R. E. Swanson, and P. J. Wiesner, "Gonococcal Ophthalmia Neonatorum: Relationship of Time of Infection to Relevant Control Measures," *JAMA*, vol. 228 (April 8, 1974).

25. J. Volk and S. J. Kraus, "Nongonococcal Urethritis: A Venereal Disease as Prevalent as Epidemic Gonorrhea," *Arch. Int. Med.*, vol. 134 (1974).

26. J. A. McChesney, A. Zedd, H. King, C. M. Russell, and J. O. Hendley, "Acute Urethritis in Male College Students," *JAMA*, vol. 226 (Oct. 1, 1973).

27. "Most Common U.S. Venereal Disease—Would You Believe Trachoma?" *Med. World News*, Oct. 4, 1974.

28. E. M. C. Dunlop, B. R. Jones, S. Darougar, and J. D. Treharne, "Chlamydia and Non-Specific Urethritis," *Brit. Med. J.*, vol. 1 (June 3, 1972).

29. G. Papaevangelou, D. Trichopoulos, T. Kremastinou, and G. Papoutsakis, "Prevalence of Hepatitis B. Antigen and Antibody in Prostitutes," *Brit. Med. J.*, vol. 1 (May 4, 1974).

30. J. Heathcote and S. Sherlock, "Spread of Acute Type-B Hepatitis in London," *Lancet*, vol. 1 (June 30, 1973).
31. K. W. M. Fulford, D. S. Dane, R. D. Catterall, R. Woof, and J. V. Denning, "Australia Antigen and Antibody among Patients Attending a Clinic for Sexually Transmitted Diseases," *Lancet*, vol. 1 (June 30, 1973).
32. "Cervical Cancer May Be Venereal," *New York Times*, April 4, 1971.
33. J. N. Goldman and M. A. Lantz, "FTA-ABS and VDRL Slide Test Reactivity in a Population of Nuns," *JAMA*, vol. 217 (July 5, 1971).
34. P. F. Sparling, "Diagnosis and Treatment of Syphilis," *New Eng. J. Med.*, vol. 284 (March 25, 1971).
35. R. D. Carr, J. W. Becker, and C. M. Carpenter, "The Biological False Positive Phenomenon in Elderly Men," *Arch. Derm.*, vol. 93 (1965).
36. S. D. Litwin and J. M. Singer, "Studies of the Incidence and Significance of Anti-Gamma Globulin Factors in the Aging," *Arthritis Rheum.*, vol. 8 (1965).
37. D. L. Tuffanelli, "Aging and False Positive Reactions for Syphilis," *Brit. J. Vener. Dis.*, vol. 42 (1966).
38. C. T. Lucas, F. Chandler Jr., J. E. Martin Jr., and J. D. Schmale, "Transfer of Gonococcal Urethritis from Man to Chimpanzee: An Animal Model for Gonorrhea," *JAMA*, vol. 216 (June 7, 1971).
39. W. Fergusson, "Observations on the Venereal Disease in Portugal," *Med. Chir. Trans.*, vol. 1 (London, 1812).
40. L. J. Goldwater, *Mercury: A History of Quicksilver* (Baltimore: York, 1972).
41. G. W. Geelhoed, "Narration: Cellini and His Syphilis—Malevolent Mercurial Cure?" *JAMA*, vol. 204 (May 13, 1968).
42. *Autobiography of Benvenuto Cellini*, trans. George Bull (Baltimore: Penguin, 1956).
43. G. Kahn, "Three Thousand Years of Mercury—A Plea for Abandonment of a Dangerous, Unproven Therapy," *Cutis.*, vol. 6 (1970).
44. J. Tongue, "An Experimental Inquiry into the Modus Operandi of Mercury, in Curing the Lues Venerea" (M.D. diss., University of Pennsylvania, 1801).
45. J. E. Moore, *Modern Treatment of Syphilis* (Springfield, Ill.: Thomas, 1933).
46. "HEW Head Assures Black M.D.'s of a Tuskegee Investigation," *Med. Tribune*, Sept. 13, 1972.

47. J. Heller, "The Syphilis Study: A 'Death Club,' " *New York Post*, Sept. 12, 1972.

48. "Comment on Tuskegee Study Varies Greatly across World," *Med. Tribune*, Oct. 25, 1972.

49. "Most Patients in PHS Study of Syphilis Were Not Treated," *Med. Tribune*, Aug. 23, 1972.

50. U.S. Department of Health, Education, and Welfare, Public Health Service, *Final Report of the Tuskegee Syphilis Study Ad Hoc Advisory Panel*, April 28, 1973.

51. B. Barber, J. J. Lally, J. L. Makarushka, and D. Sullivan, *Research on Human Subjects: Problems of Social Control in Medical Experimentation* (New York: Russell Sage Foundation, 1973).

52. H. Eagle, "The Effect of the Size of the Inoculum and the Age of the Infection on the Curative Dose of Penicillin in Experimental Infections with Streptococci, Pneumococci, and Treponema Pallidum," *J. Exp. Med.*, vol. 90 (1949).

53. O. Idsøe, T. Guthe, and R. R. Willcox, "Penicillin in the Treatment of Syphilis: The Experience of Three Decades," *Bull. WHO*, vol. 47 (1972).

54. R. D. Hahn, J. C. Cutler, A. C. Curtis, G. Gammon, A. Heyman, E. Johnwick, J. H. Stokes, H. Solomon, E. Thomas, W. Timberlake, B. Webster, and G. A. Gleeson, "Penicillin Treatment of Asymptomatic Central Nervous System Syphilis," *Arch. Derm.*, vol. 74 (1956).

55. J. B. Hardy, E. H. Oppenheimer, S. J. Ryan Jr., and R. N. Sheff, "Failure of Penicillin in a Newborn Infant with Congenital Syphilis," *JAMA*, vol. 212 (May 25, 1970).

56. "Ominous Follow-Up to Syphilis," *Med. World News*, Jan. 29, 1971.

57. H. Hooshmand, M. R. Escobar, and S. W. Kopf, "Neurosyphilis: A Study of 241 Patients," *JAMA*, vol. 219 (Feb. 7, 1972).

58. G. Hatos, "Evaluation of 460 Cases of Treated Syphilis," *Med. J. Australia*, vol. 2 (Aug. 19, 1972).

59. A. H. Rudolph and E. V. Price, "Penicillin Reactions among Patients in Venereal Disease Clinics: A Natural Survey," *JAMA*, vol. 223 (Jan. 29, 1973).

60. D. H. Robinson and D. A. Shepherd, "Single-Session, Two-Dose Therapy with Doxycycline for Gonorrhea," *Curr. Therap. Res.*, vol. 16 (1974).

61. P. J. Wiesner, H. H. Handsfield, and K. K. Holmes, "Low Antibiotic Resistance of Gonococci Causing Disseminated Infection," *New Eng. J. Med.*, vol. 288 (June 7, 1973).

62. A. Bro-Jørgensen and T. Jensen, "Gonococcal Tonsillar Infections," *Brit. Med. J.*, vol. 2 (Dec. 11, 1971).
63. N. J. Fiumara, J. D. Shinberg, E. M. Byrne, and J. Fountaine, "An Outbreak of Gonorrhea and Early Syphilis in Massachusetts," *New Eng. J. Med.*, vol. 256 (May 23, 1957).
64. N. J. Fiumara, "Gonococcal Pharyngitis," *Medical Aspects of Human Sexuality*, May 1971.
65. K. K. Holmes, D. W. Johnson, and H. J. Trostle, "An Estimate of the Risk of Men Acquiring Gonorrhea by Sexual Contact with Infected Females," *Amer. J. Epid.*, vol. 91 (1970).
66. W. F. Felton, "How Infectious Is Gonorrhea?" *Brit. Med. J.*, vol. 2 (Nov. 18, 1972).
67. J. H. Blount, "A New Approach for Gonorrhea Epidemiology," *Amer. J. Public Health*, vol. 62 (1972).
68. *Today's V.D. Control Problem—1971: A Joint Statement Published by the American Social Health Association*, Jan. 1971.
69. A. F. Marino, H. Pariser, and H. Wise, "Gonorrhea Epidemiology—Is It Worthwhile?" *Amer. J. Public Health*, vol. 62 (1972).
70. "Invisible Gonorrhea," *Newsweek*, Oct. 9, 1972.
71. "The 'Eve-Did-Syndrome': Maybe She Didn't," *JAMA*, vol. 222 (Dec. 4, 1972).
72. J. Zackler, H. Orbach, O. Brolnitsky, and M. C. Brown, "A Mass Screening Program for the Detection of Gonorrhea," *Am. J. Ob. Gyn.*, vol. 112 (1972).
73. D. W. Johnson, K. K. Holmes, P. A. Kvale, C. W. Halverson, and W. P. Hirsch, "An Evaluation of Gonorrhea Case Finding in the Chronically Infected Female," *Amer. J. Epid.*, vol. 90 (1969).
74. M. N. Bhattacharyya, A. E. Jephcott, and R. S. Morton, "Diagnosis of Gonorrhea in Women: Comparison of Sampling Sites," *Brit. Med. J.*, vol. 1 (June 30, 1973).
75. G. Moore, W. B. Pittard III, N. Mosca, and W. M. O'Brien, "Gonorrhea Detection by Urine Sediment Culture," *JAMA*, vol. 224 (June 11, 1973).
76. C. J. Stetler and A. R. Moritz, *Doctor and Patient and the Law* (St. Louis: Mosby, 1962).
77. Simonson v. Swenson, 104 Neb 224, 177 N.W. 831 (1920).
78. R. A. Vonderlehr and J. R. Heller Jr., *The Control of Venereal Disease* (New York: Reynal and Hitchcock, 1946).
79. "Gonorrhea Vaccine Fails in Inuvik Trial," *Hospital Tribune*, Sept. 17, 1973.

80. J. A. Yacenda, "Survey of VD Knowledge among Young People," *Health Services Reports*, vol. 87 (1972).
81. "V.D.: The Epidemic," *Newsweek*, Jan. 24, 1972.
82. *New York Times*, Aug. 26, 1973.
83. L. Baumgartner, "Syphilis Eradication—A Plan for Action Now," *Proc. World Forum on Syphilis and Other Treponematoses* (Public Health Service Publication no. 997; Washington, D.C.: Government Printing Office, 1964).
84. R. H. Kampmeier, "The Matter of Venereal Disease in 1971," *Ann. Int. Med.*, vol. 75 (1971).
85. P. G. Boysen, "Venereal Disease Education," *JAMA*, vol. 221 (Sept. 11, 1972).
86. "Medical News," *MD*, June 1971.
87. "Gonorrhea at Record Rate: Syphilis Highest since '50," *American Medical News*, April 2, 1973.

SUGGESTED ADDITIONAL READINGS

Historical References

Fracastor, Hieronymus. *Syphilis.* (A translation.) St. Louis: Philmar, 1911.
The sixteenth-century poem from which the disease got its name.
Goldwater, Leonard J. *Mercury: A History of Quicksilver.* Baltimore: York, 1972.
A scholarly and interesting monograph by one of the world's experts on mercury.
Parran, Thomas, M.D. *Shadow on the Land: Syphilis.* New York: Reynal and Hitchcock, 1937.
A blockbuster of a book in its day, written by the man who finally began to rip away the secrecy and shame that cloaked public thinking about syphilis.
Vonderlehr, R. A., and J. R. Heller Jr., *The Control of Venereal Disease.* New York: Reynal and Hitchcock, 1946.
Out of date, but folksy and entertaining.

General References

Neumann, Hans H., M.D., with Sylvia Simmons. *The Straight Story on VD.* New York: Warner, 1973.
A question-and-answer book about VD. Has a good list of places to call, visit, or write to for information or help.
Rosebury, Theodore. *Microbes and Morals.* New York: Viking, 1971.

A splendid book by a well-known microbiologist who is also a fine science writer. Especially good on the historical and literary aspects of VD.

VD Blues. New York: Avon, 1973.

The original script for the successful TV show, plus an edited transcript of the New York hot-line show that followed. Also has a list of places to call for information.

Biological and Medical References

Medical Clinics of North America. *Symposium on Syphilis and Other Venereal Diseases,* ed. John B. Youmans, M.D. Philadelphia: Saunders, 1964.

A number of excellent articles on different aspects of VD, all written by experts.

Thomas, Evan W., M.D. *Syphilis: Its Course and Management.* New York: Macmillan, 1949.

Also a bit dated, but a fine book nevertheless, detailing the experience of one of the largest and best VD clinics in the world.

Turner, Thomas Bourne, and David H. Hollander. *Biology of the Treponematoses.* Geneva: World Health Organization, 1957.

For those who want more scientific information on the laboratory investigation of infectious treponemes. Not easy going for laymen.

U.S. Department of Health, Education, and Welfare. *Proceedings of World Forum on Syphilis and Other Treponematoses.* Public Health Service Publication no. 997. Washington, D.C.: Government Printing Office, 1962.

A big book covering many aspects of these international diseases.

_____. *Syphilis: A Synopsis.* Public Health Service Publication no. 1660. Washington, D.C.: Government Printing Office, 1968.

_____. *Syphilis: Modern Diagnosis and Treatment.* Public Health Service Publication no. 1961. Washington, D.C.: Government Printing Office, 1961.

Two books with many good colored photos of syphilitic lesions.

Glossary

anaphylaxis	an extreme hypersensitivity, seen in both animals and man; manifested by dramatic and dangerous effects which can be fatal
aneurysm	a localized dilation of an arterial wall
antibiotic	a substance, derived from a mold or bacterium, that kills, or inhibits the growth of, other microorganisms
antibody	a modified protein produced by the body in response to an antigen
antigen	a material that stimulates antibody production when brought into contact with the appropriate body tissues
arsenical	a compound containing an arsenic salt; these drugs were once a mainstay of antisyphilitic treatment
Candida albicans	a yeastlike organism, ordinarily benign, that can produce infection of the lungs, heart, skin, vagina, vulva, and penis; also called *Monilia albicans*—hence the diseases it causes are called either candidiasis or moniliasis
cardiovascular	relating to the circulation, or to the heart and blood vessels

151

chancre

the lesion of primary syphilis; begins as a hard, dull red, painless bump which later breaks down to form an ulcer

chancroid

one of the less common venereal diseases; characterized by multiple painful ulcers on the penis or vulva

Clutton's joints

a manifestation of congenital syphilis; consists of painless joint swellings, especially of the knees

congenital syphilis

syphilis acquired by the fetus in the uterus before birth

conjunctivitis

inflammation of the delicate, transparent membrane covering the exposed surface of the eyeball and the inner surface of the eyelids

darkfield microscopy

visualization of an object under the microscope by faint light reflected onto the object from the sides; used to see live spirochetes

diplococcal

referring to more or less round bacteria that occur in pairs; the gonococcus, pneumococcus, and meningococcus are examples of diplococci

epidemiology

the science dealing with the incidence, spread, and control of disease

epidydimis

an elongated cordlike structure along the posterior border of the testis

fallopian tube

the long slender tube extending from the uterus to the region of the ovary on the same side

false positive

a test that falsely suggests the presence of disease

fluorescein

a yellow or red dye that fluoresces with a bright yellow-green color in alkaline solution

FTA-ABS test

the fluorescent treponemal antibody absorption blood test for diagnosis of syphilis

general paresis	a form of tertiary syphilis characterized by dementia and delusions of grandeur
gonococcus	the cause of gonorrhea; a kidney-shaped diplococcus whose scientific name is *Neisseria gonorrhoeae*
granuloma inguinale	one of the less common venereal diseases, caused by the "Donovan body"; characterized by lesions on the groin and genitals that become raised, red, and velvety and bleed easily
gumma	one form of tertiary syphilis; a soft gummy tumor
hepatitis	inflammation of the liver
herpes progenitalis	an inflammatory disease characterized by small blisters, in clusters, on the genitals; thought by some to be related to cervical cancer
Herxheimer reaction	a rarely occurring explosive inflammatory or allergic response around tissue spirochetes as a result of treatment; also called the Jarisch-Herxheimer reaction
Hutchinson's teeth	notched and narrow-edged permanent incisors; a sign of congenital syphilis
infectious mononucleosis	a usually benign disease characterized by sore throat, rash, and enlargement of the spleen and lymph nodes
IUD	a device inserted into the uterus to prevent conception
keratitis	inflammation of the cornea
Kolmer test	a diagnostic blood test for syphilis
lichen planus	an inflammatory skin disease characterized by wide flat bumps in circumscribed patches
lymphogranuloma venereum	one of the less common venereal diseases; can lead to elephantiasis of the scrotum or labia and to rectal strictures
meningitis	inflammation of the membranous envelopes surrounding the brain and spinal cord

meningococcus	one cause of meningitis; a relative of the gonococcus, which it closely resembles
meningovascular	one type of secondary syphilis, caused by involvement of the blood vessels of the meninges
Monilia	old name for the genus of fungi now called *Candida* (see Candida albicans)
mulberry molars	a manifestation of congenital syphilis; molar teeth with irregular crowns, whose enamel appears like an aggregated mass of globules
mycoplasma	a genus of so-called pleuropneumonia-like organisms (PPLO); cause a variety of illnesses, including so-called atypical pneumonia and possibly urethritis
Neisseria gonorrhoeae	*see* gonococcus
nephritis	inflammation of the kidneys
pinta	a tropical disease that resembles syphilis in its manifestations; spread by skin contact and caused by a spirochete identical in appearance to the one that causes syphilis
pityriasis rosea	a skin disease characterized by pinkish oval patches with a crinkled, dry epidermis; lesions appear on the back, arms, legs, and thighs
placenta	a cakelike organ in the uterus, through which the fetus receives nourishment from the mother via the umbilical cord
prophylaxis	prevention of disease
prostate	the male gland that surrounds the urethra and the bladder neck
prozone phenomenon	a paradoxical lab result wherein serum with a high agglutinin titer fails to cause agglutination in low dilution
psoriasis	a skin disease characterized by silvery gray, scaly, shiny red plaques on the arms, legs, and scalp

reagin	a type of antibody; important in blood tests for syphilis
rheumatoid arthritis	a common form of chronic arthritis, characterized by symmetrically swollen, red, tender joints
rheumatoid factor	a substance found in the serum of many patients with rheumatoid arthritis
ringworm	popular name for ring-shaped, pigmented bumps with blisters or scaling; caused by members of the fungus family
saprophyte	an organism living on dead or decaying organic matter
scabies	a contagious skin disease caused by the itch mite, which bores beneath the skin, forming burrows and causing intense itching
serological	relating to blood serum
spirochete	a corkscrew-shaped microorganism
tabes dorsalis	a form of tertiary syphilis affecting the spinal cord
titer	the quantity of a substance which will react with a given volume or amount of another substance
treponema	a genus of spirochete causing syphilis, yaws, and pinta; also contains nonpathogenic members
TPI test	the treponema immobilization test; used for diagnosing syphilis
Treponema pallidum	the organism that causes syphilis
Trichomonas	a genus of parasitic protozoa; common cause of vaginitis
urethra	a membranous canal carrying urine from the bladder to the exterior of the body
VDRL test	a commonly used blood test for diagnosing syphilis
venereologist	a physician specializing in the diagnosis and treatment of venereal disease
vulvovaginitis	inflammation of the vulva and vagina

Wassermann test   the oldest diagnostic test for syphilis

yaws   a tropical disease spread by skin contact and causing lesions in the skin and bones; caused by a spirochete identical in appearance to the one causing syphilis

Index

158   *Index*